Doctors Guide to **End Your**

THYROID
PROBLEMS

Discover what your Doctor is missing

Dr. Tom Sladic DC, CNS

The information and recommendations in this book are not intended as a substitute for professional medical advice. It is the sole responsibility of the user to determine if the procedures are appropriate. This author cannot be held responsible for the information or any inadvertent errors resulting from attempting any of the protocols. The nutritional supplements mentioned are not intended to be used to diagnose, treat, cure or prevent disease. This book should not be used as replacement for any medical treatment.

CONTENTS

Chapter 6:
What Can You Do To Start Feeling Better?

Chapter 7:

My name is Dr. Tom Sladic.
I have a private practice in the State of Michigan. I am a member of the Institute for Functional Medicine and the American College of Nutrition. I am a Certified Nutrition Specialist and Chiropractic Physician. I wrote this book to help those suffering from hypothyroidism get the answers and help they need. I have helped hundreds of patients get better and I wanted to share my strategies with those who continue to suffer. This book is meant to be a guide so that you can get some insight into what might be happening in your own situation. The solutions are a completely natural approach that delivers consistently excellent results.

I will show you what I do for my patients so that they get well. I will also share some examples of different cases at the end of this book. You might find that you could benefit from some advanced testing and some blood tests that you may not have heard of before. You will get to know the diets and supplements I use for my patients in different cases. If you find yourself falling into a certain category, you'll know exactly what to do.

I suggest that you work with a professional in regard to the nutritional protocols and be sure to get high-quality supplements. Many of my patients are on medications prior to seeing me and they continue to take these as we work together. Do not stop taking any medications that you are prescribed. Over time, you will notice that you start to feel much better as your health improves. At that point, your doctor may reduce the amount of medication you are taking. I will also share with you the type of blood tests I perform, which you can use to monitor your health.

When your thyroid is not working properly, a number of things can go wrong with you. One of the biggest complaints is fatigue. Added weight gain, even when on a low calorie diet, is another symptom.

I have patients who eat 1,200 calories a day doing a 6-month boot camp and they haven't lost a single pound. In such cases, there's obviously something wrong and it is not your genetics. Some other symptoms of thyroid problems are: morning headaches which wear off as the day progresses, depression, constipation and sensitivity to cold.

If your hands are freezing and you're cold during mid-summer, you have poor blood circulation, numbness in your hands and feet, muscle cramps, you have colds and are sickly all the time, wounds which heal slowly, you require excessive amounts of sleep to function properly, you suffer digestive problems, have itchy skin, dry brittle hair, hair loss and a loss of a portion of your eyebrows, leg swelling and edema, there is high probability that you have some thyroid dysfunction.

Every cell in your body has thyroid receptors. So, if your thyroid is not functioning, there are many, many different parts of your body that are going to be affected. One of them is bone metabolism. The thyroid secretes something called calcitonin which is responsible for laying down bone.

Many patients who have had thyroid problems for a long time end up on osteoporosis medication.

Anemia is another red flag. Your thyroid is responsible for producing stomach acid. When you have a thyroid problem, stomach acid production goes down. Consequently, B12 and iron absorption becomes difficult. That can lead to anemia. Unfortunately, many patients end up taking antacids to correct this - which only makes the problem worse.

Body heat and night sweats: The thyroid is the thermostat of your body. It controls your body temperature. Indeed, your body temperature has a lot to do with your thyroid, estrogen imbalance and adrenal glands. If you're sweating a lot, that's an adrenal problem. Supporting the adrenal glands will get things in balance, including menopausal symptoms. In some cases, we use a temperature graph to differentiate what the problem is to monitor progress (See Chapter 6).

Another problem is estrogen metabolism. When you have hypothyroidism, the liver detox pathways will slow down, especially detox pathway number two (which is responsible for getting estrogen out of your body). In turn, estrogen will build up in your bloodstream and gets stored in fat tissue. I'm sure you are aware that high levels of estrogen are very bad. It can cause cancer, ovarian cysts and a number of other complications. This book will tell you exactly how to detoxify the liver which is only done after first addressing the thyroid.

Gastrointestinal dysfunction: Slow intestinal tract motility can cause constipation. More importantly, the waste and toxic material that sits in your gut for many days can cause an overgrowth of bad bacteria. This is called dysbiosis and will begin to negatively impact your health and lead to numerous problems. You should be having bowel movement on a daily basis.

Gallbladder: One of the biggest issues I see with thyroid patients is that many have already had their gallbladder removed. Your liver and gallbladder become congested because you have low thyroid symptoms (slow function) and cannot detox things. The gallbladder becomes inflamed and possibly congested with stones; you go in for surgery and it gets removed.

Progesterone production: Progesterone is secreted during the second half of your cycle. So, if you feel miserable during the two weeks leading up to your period, you very well could have a problem with progesterone. In addition, you need a nice progesterone surge that stimulates TPO production - which helps your body produce thyroid hormones. So, when you have an imbalance, you're going to have all these symptoms: heavy bleeding, difficulty in losing weight, irritability and headaches.

Fat burning: This is an easy one to figure out. Your thyroid runs your metabolism. If your metabolism is slow, you're not going to be able to burn body fat at all.

Insulin and glucose metabolism: Glucose is not going to be absorbed by the cells like it's supposed to and you're going to start gaining a lot of weight. You tend to have fatigue after meals. You may also have the hypoglycemic pattern which includes headaches and brain fog. When you're not absorbing glucose properly, you may experience brain fog, fatigue, difficulty in concentrating.

Healthy Cholesterol Levels: Everyone is concerned about cholesterol these days; but I'll tell you: cholesterol is managed by your liver. Your liver manages the amount of cholesterol in the bloodstream. If you have a low thyroid, your liver is going to be congested and you may have an excessive amount of fatty acids in the blood. So, you'll have a high amount of total cholesterol as a result of hypothyroidism. By addressing the thyroid, cholesterol levels fall to normal ranges.

From what I just mentioned, you can see how many different systems of your body are affected when you have thyroid dysfunction. The good news is that by addressing the cause you will feel a dramatic change in so many different areas, since every cell in your body has thyroid receptors.

Can you tell me why you have a thyroid problem? Why are you on thyroid medication? What's wrong with you? Not many patients can answer these questions because nobody has given them an answer. To uncover a problem, you have to first acknowledge and understand it. Why is the thyroid not working properly and what is causing its dysfunction? Let's start by understanding how thyroid hormone is made and delivered, using the diagram below.

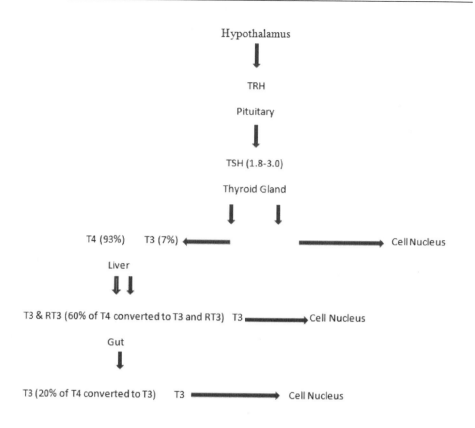

We start with the hypothalamus and pituitary gland. The hypothalamus releases TRH (Thyrotropin releasing hormone) to signal the pituitary gland to release TSH (thyroid stimulating hormone). If you have thyroid problems, TSH is one of the tests that your doctor will run. The ideal range should be 1.8 - 3.0. Low levels of serotonin and dopamine can affect the hypothalamus. Also, physical, chemical, psychological and environmental stress can affect the pituitary. You may have some problems with either the pituitary or the hypothalmus. This could be true if your TSH is between 0.8 and 1.8, you are not on thyroid hormone and you have the symptoms of hypothyroidism. It's important to understand that the thyroid doesn't secrete TSH. It is the pituitary gland secreting TSH to instruct the thyroid to produce some hormones. Your thyroid gland produces two hormones: T4 and T3.

T4 has 4 molecules of iodine and T3 has 3 molecules

of iodine. Your body produces 93% of T4 and 7% T3. T4 is inactive and T3 is active. It's important to understand that since T4 is inactive, it must be converted to active T3 to be used by the body. Sixty percent of T4 is converted in the liver, 20% in the gut and the remaining portion is converted in the muscles and other cells. So, T4 actually becomes T3. T4 and T3 are delivered to the cells by a protein called thyroid binding globulin (TBG). They get transported to the cells. Eventually, they get to the cell receptor site where the cell accepts T3. Once T3 gets into the cell, it signals the DNA, runs the metabolism and performs other essential functions. That said, thyroid dysfunction can occur at any of these points. It is important that bloodwork check all mentioned factors. Tests are further discussed in Chapter 4.

Now that you understand some of the basic mechanisms, let's explore some common problems. First and foremost, you must be screened for an autoimmune disease called Hashimoto's. If you have an autoimmune condition, your symptoms will wax and wane, which means that some days you feel good and some days you feel bad. It just keeps going back and forth. In addition, your TSH is always jumping around and your doctor is constantly adjusting your thyroid hormone. These are just some clues that I often pick up. Both TPO and Thyroglobulin antibodies need to be tested to confirm that you have this condition.

Why is this important? If your immune system is attacking your thyroid, the thyroid gland will be impaired as it will not be able to produce any hormone. To help the thyroid, in such a case, the attack must be stopped completely. This is a **very** important concept to understand. Please read it again. To simplify: the thyroid gland is not working properly because it is being attacked by the immune system. What is the solution? To restore proper function, the attack must be stopped. It's that simple. I can say that this is missed or not properly managed in at least 60% of the patients I see. Most patients have not even heard of Hashimoto's and have never been tested. In my practice, if you have an autoimmune condition, it changes the course of care you get. The immune system must be managed in order to help the patient. I will give you some strategies for this in Chapter 3.

Odds are that your medical doctor may not have performed this test and it may not be important to them. You see, it doesn't change their treatment which involves thyroid hormone replacement (Synthroid). Their goal is to get your TSH value between 1-5 and you are then considered fixed! However, to get to the root cause of your problem, you must address and manage the autoimmune condition (Hashimoto's). That's one very common

problem I see and one reason you continue to suffer. An autoimmune disease is a condition where the body attacks its own tissue. With time, the tissue destruction becomes permanent. This should be the first thing to screen for and manage.

There is another autoimmune disease called Grave's Disease (hyperactive thyroid). The symptoms include: insomnia, heart palpitations, inward trembling, weight loss, anxiety, increased pulse rate at rest and night sweats. Grave's is not as common as Hashimoto's; however, it can be life threatening as it can cause cardiovascular problems. It's also common for a patient with Hashimoto's to have some hyperthyroid symptoms as they sometimes swing from hypothyroid to hyperthyroid. You may not have Grave's but if your TSH is out of range on the low end (below 0.5) and your T4 and T3 are high, you may need to run the antibody test TSI or TSAab in order to rule out Grave's. If your TSH is low and you are on thyroid hormone, your doctor will most likely adjust your dose since that would be the cause of the low TSH. Grave's is also an immune system problem that needs to be managed. It should be co-managed with a cardiol-ogist due to the cardiovascular implications. Again, it is not as common as Hashimoto's and you may not have Grave's.

I often see a group of patients who have had their thyroid removed or destroyed with radioactive iodine as a result of having been diagnosed with Grave's. Consequently, they must be on thyroid hormone for life. Most of them suffer with symptoms of hypothyroidism, including weight gain, dry skin, hair loss, fatigue and lack of energy. However, by addressing the immune system, we can reduce the symptoms in many of these cases. Destroying or removing the gland did not address the underlying autoimmune disease. It is not going to just go away. To keep it simple: **autoimmune disease requires repair of the immune system**.

The goal is to deliver thyroid hormone to the cell nucleus (as depicted on the diagram). Autoimmune thyroid disease is most likely Hashimoto's attacking your thyroid gland. The problem occurs at the level of the thyroid gland and the solution is to address the attack. The common causes of and management strategies for autoimmune disease will be discussed later in this book.

Next on the list of possible thyroid dysfunction is thyroid conversion. If we refer back to our diagram, you will notice that the thyroid produces about 93% T4 hormone which is inactive. T4 is converted to the active form T3 throughout the body, predominantly by the liver which converts 60% of the T4 to T3. The balance of the conversion next occurs in the gut/intestine where 20% is converted and the remaining conversion occurs in other tissues and cells. To see if conversion is a problem, your T3 and free T3 levels are examined via blood tests. If the number is low, then it is possible that you may have an issue with conversion. I first check

the liver enzymes ALT and AST to see if they are in the functional range of 10-26. Next, I check the gut for infections, parasites, yeast and dysbiosis (an imbalance of gut bacteria). To help with conversion issues, I would proceed with correcting the liver detox pathways and repair gut function. These strategies are discussed in Chapter 6.

Thyroid resistance is another common problem. You have probably heard of insulin resistance, when the cells are resistant to insulin, which leads to diabetes. With thyroid resistance, the cells are resistant to thyroid hormone and do not allow it to enter the cell - most commonly resulting from toxins and inflammation. I check homocysteine levels along with C-reactive protein to measure inflammation. Lack of good fatty acids in the blood can also cause cellular resistance. I use essential fatty acids or fish oil to help solve this issue. Testing for inflammation and establishing whether all thyroid numbers are within range will determine whether thyroid resistance is a problem.

Anemia is another consideration. If you have anemia, you will have cold hands, fatigue and may have an urge to chew on ice cubes. When testing for anemia, be sure to also have your ferritin levels checked since ferritin is the stored form of iron which is usually neglected. It is important to be checked for uterine fibroids or cysts since they can very well cause anemia. If you are anemic, your cells are lacking oxygen. With no oxygen, the thyroid will not function properly. Check iron, TIBC/saturation and ferritin.

The adrenal glands are intimately connected to thyroid function. It is a must to check them as they can hamper normal thyroid function. The adrenal glands produce Cortisol and DHEA. Patients with adrenal issues tend to have lower blood sugar levels, suffer from fatigue, headaches and have sleep disturbances. When a person is under chronic stress, the adrenals will release extra Cortisol. When this happens, the connection between the hypothalamus and pituitary becomes weakened which can affect TSH production. Adrenal stress can also hamper the conversion of T4 to T3 causing cellular resistance to thyroid hormone. One of the biggest stressors to the adrenal glands is dysglycemia (blood sugar swings). This is created by taking sporadic meals, skipping breakfast and eating foods that are high in sugar. The best way to determine if you have a problem with your adrenal glands is to do a salivary test called Adrenal Stress Index (ASI). It measures Cortisol levels throughout the day and will also determine if you have a healthy Cortisol-to-DHEA ratio. Some symptoms of adrenal dysfunction include: trouble sleeping, morning fatigue, afternoon crashes, salt cravings, headaches, and excessive sweating.

Adrenal glands must be checked as they could be causing your thyroid problems. The adrenals can also be affected by food allergies, blood sugar (as previously mentioned), gut dysfunction and anemia.

It is amazing how much sugar people eat. Fast foods and high carbohydrate diets are part of the lifestyle for so many. For instance, breakfast might be coffee with double sugar, a bagel or a muffin, juice and/or a candy bar. I remember being at the checkout line at Home Depot and noticing someone grabbing a Mountain Dew and a candy bar out of the vending machine at 7:30 a.m. for breakfast. It was then that I realized how big of a problem we have. Obesity rates and diabetes (including diabetes in children) are on the rise. Dysglycemia happens when the body loses its ability to keep blood sugar stable. The cells require oxygen and a steady supply of ATP for energy. Blood sugar problems will affect ATP. This in turns weakens the gut and immune system (which makes you susceptible to Hashimoto's), causing hormonal imbalances. Excessive hormones will cause the liver detox pathways to become clogged which can cause hair loss. This can impact normal thyroid function. Fasting blood sugar should be between 80 and 100 and your A1C should be below 5.7. People with hypoglycemic tendencies will have fasting sugars below 80 and LDH below 140.

The GI tract and gut health must be evaluated including: barrier integrity (leaky gut), hypochlorhydria (stomach acid), dysbiosis and parasitic/bacterial infections. Leaky gut, also known as intestinal permeability, is a condition whereby the gut barrier is weakened. This affects nutrient absorption. The thyroid gland requires Vitamins A and D, zinc, selenium and tyrosine to function properly. When absorption of nutrients is impaired, the gland will malfunction. In the case of leaky gut, when the barrier is weakened, undigested foods wastes and toxins can enter the bloodstream which bombards the immune system, setting the stage for autoimmune disease (Hashimoto's). I use a blood test from Cyrex Labs to test for leaky gut.

Hypochlorhydria sets the stage for low stomach acid. Having low stomach acid creates a situation where food is not broken down. A low acidic environment becomes a breeding ground for infections. It is important to be screened for H-pylori since it can also be an antigen which could contribute to autoimmune disease. If you are taking Prilosec or any form of antacids, you **must** fix this situation as it will create health problems leading to osteoporosis since antacids deplete mineral absorption, have an increased risk of intestinal infection, deplete the absorption of Vitamin B12 and increase your risk of developing food allergies. I check total protein, albumin and globulin in these situations. If these are high or low, I suspect hypochlorhydria. These blood values are provided for your reference in Chapter 5.

Dysbiosis is an imbalance of good bacteria and bad bacteria within the intestinal tract. The microbiome is a new frontier in research. There are over 400 species of bacteria in the colon. It is believed that 60-80% of your immune system resides in the gut. It is easy to see that if you have a dysfunctional bacterial environment it can lead to autoimmune diseases. The most common culprits are antibiotics and a diet high in sugar which will disrupt the bacterial colonies. As you will note in our diagram, 20% of T4 is converted into T3 in the gut. Transit time is another issue to consider with GI dysfunction. You should have a bowel movement every 18-24 hours. If you are not clearing toxins, excess hormones and wastes from the body, delivery of thyroid hormone to the cells is affected. I typically use stool tests to check for infections and/or GI function. If you have IBS symptoms and have digestive complaints, you should suspect problems with the GI tract. Chapter 6 addresses how to correct these issues.

Tried Everything And You Are Not Getting Better?

a) hyroid Replacement - Did you know that over 200 medications contain gluten including thyroid hormone? Thyroid supplements and thyroid hormone replacement can contain modified food starch including cornstarch and gluten. If you have a sensitivity to these, you will be making your condition worse.

b) Stress - Emotional stressors create inflammation throughout the body. Inflammation can keep you from getting well. Be sure to create a healthy emotional environment for yourself.

c) Diet - Not following your diet 100%. If you are on a gluten-free diet, are you still consuming gluten every once in a while? Cheating on your diet will sabotage your results.

d) Wrong Supplements - If you have Hashimoto's, you have an imbalance in your immune system. You are either TH1 or TH2 dominant. Ideally, we want a balance between TH1 and TH2. So, if you are taking supplements that increase TH1 or TH2, you will get worse. For example, coffee is a TH1 stimulator. If you are TH1 dominant, you will be increasing the imbalance by drinking coffee. Refer to the section on autoimmunity to determine if you are TH1 or TH2 dominant.

e) Gluten-free is not always safe - You might be reacting

to gluten-free foods including corn, rice, potato, casein and oats. It is best to perform a test from Cyrex Labs to see what is safe and what is not.

f) Ignoring blood sugar - Eating sweets or sugary drinks throughout the day can trigger insulin surges. This creates an inflammatory response and will keep you from getting well. In addition, skipping meals or going hours without eating will also create problems.

g) Poor attitude - People who are not willing to put in the time and effort to get well. If you believe you will never get well, you will never get well. Everyone has excuses. The person who has the will to succeed will succeed.

h) Not managing autoimmunity - Many patients are concerned with changing their thyroid medication. If you have autoimmune disease, your concern should be managing the autoimmune attack on the thyroid gland. Your thyroid medication does **not** fix autoimmune disease. It only replaces the deficient hormone. The very reason your thyroid is not working is due to your immune system attacking it. You will never get better if this is not managed.

i) Worried about thyroid supplements and ignoring any underlying causes - Hidden gut

infections, gut function, anemia, food sensitivities, heavy metal toxicity, adrenal and hormones and inflammation.

Understanding Autoimmune Disease (Hashimoto's)

If you have a thyroid problem, it is imperative that you get tested for Hashimoto's through TPO and Thyroglobulin antibodies. In this chapter, we will explore Hashimoto's disease.

With Hashimoto's, our immune system is mistakenly attacking the thyroid. It is making auto antibodies. It is not distinguishing between 'self' and 'non-self'.

Your immune system has two responses: the TH1 and the TH2 response. When a person has an autoimmune disease, one of these systems is 'hyper-firing' and is dominant. Balancing this system goes a long way toward reducing symptoms:

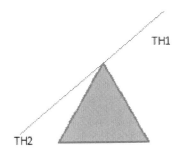
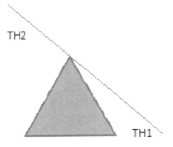

Our bodies have natural barriers to protect us from toxins and pathogens:

- Skin (enzymes)
- Lungs (coughing/sneezing)
- Eyes (tears)
- Mucus (respiratory tract to trap pathogens)
- Gut Flora (to compete with pathogens)

Also, our white blood cells respond to invaders in special ways. You can have a TH1 response or a TH2 response. The TH1 response is the first line of defense and is an innate response to kill invaders. The TH2 response is an identification response that labels the invader so that the body will identify it for purposes of future exposure. In simple terms, a TH2 response will put labels and tags on things in order for the TH1 system to attack it. The more out of balance this system becomes, the more tissue destruction will occur.

There are possibilities for this to occur:

1. The immune system is imbalanced due to an 'invader'; i.e., a chronic infection (bacterial, viral, mold, etc.), an infection in the gut, food sensitivities, environmental toxins or Leaky Gut Syndrome.

2. The immune system is out of balance due to chronic stressors. This includes: chronic inflammation from a poor diet, unstable blood sugar, bad adrenal glands, hormone imbalances, post-pregnancy and low Vitamin D.

TH1 or TH2 Dominance and Appropriate Supplements:

**Things that stimulate the TH1 response:
(Take if you are TH2 Dominant)**

Echinacea

Garlic

Vitamin C

Immune Stimulants:

Licorice root (Glycyrrhiza)

Astragalus

Beta-glucan mushroom

Maitake mushroom (Grifola frondosa)

Lemon balm (Melissa officinalis)

Things that stimulate the TH2 response:
(Take if you are TH1 Dominant)

Caffeine

Green tea

Grape seed extract

Herbal barks (Cramp bark, Pine bark, White Willow bark)

Lycopene

Resveratrol

Pycnogenol

If you take anything listed above and it makes you feel worse, it would indicate dominance. For example, if echinacea or anything that stimulates a TH1 response makes you feel sick or bad, you would be TH1 dominant. You would then avoid everything that stimulates a TH1 response and take products that stimulate a TH2 response in order to balance the TH1/TH2 system. Conversely, if caffeine or anything that stimulates a TH2 response makes you feel worse, you would then avoid anything that stimulates a TH2 response and take products that stimulate a TH1 response.

NOTE:
If you are not able to detect any noticeable differences, fish oil, Vitamin D, glutathione and nitric oxide will help balance the systems.

Another clue for determining TH1 or TH2 dominance is to evaluate how you felt during a pregnancy, if applicable. During pregnancy, the body becomes TH2 dominant. After pregnancy, a shift to TH1 balance should occur. If you felt great during pregnancy, it is possible that you are TH1 dominant. If you felt horrible while pregnant, it is possible that you are TH2 dominant.

The challenge to managing autoimmune thyroid conditions is balancing the immune system and removing any triggers including chronic infections (bacterial, viral, mold), gut infections, food sensitivities and environmental toxins.

The next step is to fix leaky gut syndrome and strengthen the immune system. A large part of your immune system (50-80%) resides in the gut. Six months of quality probiotics dosed at 100 billion per day, along with immunoglobulins, will also help. It is important to check for chronic inflammation from a poor diet using blood tests including C-Reactive protein and homocysteine. Lastly, correct unstable blood sugar, dysfunctional adrenal glands, hormone imbalances and low Vitamin D.

Hormones

In this section, I want to share some information on the hormones estrogen and progesterone since they can impact or mimic some thyroid symptoms. A general rule for hormone issues is that they usually result from a downstream problem - often unstable blood sugar and adrenals. Fifty percent of hormone problems can be solved by correcting adrenal function.

Some symptoms of female hormone imbalance are: weight gain, fatigue, depression, low sex drive, crying easily, mood swings, cravings for sweets, PMS, hot flashes, night sweats, irritability, irrational thoughts, anxiety, dry skin, hair loss, osteoporosis, fluid retention, infertility and irregular cycles.

Factors that can contribute to hormone imbalance include: adrenal gland dysfunction (Cortisol and DHEA), unstable blood sugar (insulin surges), inflammation, poor gut function, anemia, poor liver function and poor thyroid function.

The female cycle has basically two halves. The first half is estrogen based (follicular phase) and the second half is progesterone based (luteal phase). Day one is the first day of bleeding. Both estrogen and progesterone will be low on day one. Prompted by FSH, estrogen levels begin to rise promoting growth of the follicle. A peak in estrogen causes stimulation of LH to cause the egg to erupt from the follicle which becomes the corpus luteum. The corpus luteum becomes a source of progesterone. Progesterone levels begin to fall around Day 28 joining low levels of estrogen and menstruation begins and the cycle continues.

All hormones come from cholesterol. Cholesterol converts to pregnenolone. Pregnenolone can convert to DHEA and progesterone. Progesterone can convert to Cortisol. If Cortisol is low, the body will shift pregnenolone to make Cortisol which will cause low progesterone. DHEA can convert to estrogen. Some practitioners will use pregnenolone to try and boost progesterone. This is not always the case as it may not go straight to progesterone. However, DHEA can boost estrogen. Vaginal dryness is a classic sign of low estrogen and DHEA can help with this. There are other hormones involved in this pathway including Androstenedione, Testosterone and DHT.

The best way to check for hormone production is salivary testing. If you are a cycling female, a 28-day test is available that will plot hormone production through your entire cycle giving valuable insight into what needs to be addressed. In perimenopausal women, hormone spikes and drops can be erratic. If you are menopausal, an alternate one-day test is available. Always check Cortisol levels with this test as it is a salivary test also. Blood tests do not pick up free fraction hormones. For example, if you use creams, hormones get stored in fat cells and a blood test will not show this.

There are three stages to hormone imbalance:

1. Poor distribution - Producing enough but not producing at the right time. One of the most common problems is that progesterone drops off too quickly. The second common problem is that estrogen spikes too soon,

causing a spike in Progesterone at the wrong time and you won't ovulate.

2. Low output- This will cause menopause

3. Timing problems- causing problems with ovulation.

Here are some key points to be aware of:

- Classic PMS is an early drop off of progesterone.

- Progesterone production slows during a woman's early 30's and estrogen does not slow until perimenopause. Progesterone drops to about 75%. Estrogen dominates due to progesterone deficiency.

- A dip in estrogen or a dip in progesterone can cause migraine headaches. Adrenal exhaustion can create a state of estrogen dominance.

- Your progesterone is dominant during pregnancy.

- When estrogen is unopposed, you will get a thickening of the uterine lining.

- T3 is a huge stimulant to the corpus luteum which creates progesterone. Check for low T3.

- The pill decreases LH which creates no corpus luteum and no progesterone. You can become estrogen dominant from birth control pills.

- A good ratio of Progesterone to Estrogen is 40:1

- The adrenal glands are responsible for 30% of hormone production in pre-menopausal women

- Progesterone increases bone production. Therefore, low levels will cause osteoporosis.

Symptoms of excess estrogen include: Breast swelling and tenderness, fibroids, cystic ovaries, heavy/irregular periods, weight gain, mood swings, craving for sweets, water retention, low libido, anxiety, headaches and hair loss.

These symptoms are also the same if you are progesterone

deficient as it makes you estrogen dominant. If progesterone falls and estrogen remains the same, you are estrogen dominant by default. It is common today for most women to be estrogen dominant as we live in a world where we are exposed to xenoestrogens which readily convert to estrogen. This will cause women to not ovulate, which seems to be a more common problem today.

If you are preparing for pregnancy, then it's important that you begin taking care of yourself at least 3-6 months prior. Most people start taking care of themselves once they know they are pregnant. Adopt good dietary, nutritional and lifestyle habits and avoid toxins. Do not perform any type of detox for at least 3 months prior to conception.

To address infertility issues, run the 28-day salivary hormone test to pinpoint any issues. The saliva test will show any hormone production drops or timing issues. Correct any adrenal exhaustion and liver issues. Many of these people can also be gluten intolerant and have digestive tract infections. In addition, the male partner should be checked and his overall health optimized, not just his sperm.

Solutions for Hormone Problems

Most doctors and patients will want to skip steps and just start taking hormones. Remember, we are exposed to xenoestrogens so it is highly likely that most women are estrogen dominant considering the fact that progesterone production slows at age 30. Therefore, since the adrenal glands are responsible for 30-50% of hormone production, they must be strong. Secondly, estrogen is cleared in the gut. If you have an imbalance of gut bacteria, estrogen will not be cleared from the body and will recirculate. A good probiotic along with correction of any yeast or parasite issues will help. Fiber and Indol3carbinol will help. I have used a product from Designs for Health called DIM. The liver needs to be supported as it is also responsible for clearing estrogen. Some women will feel better just from clearing extra estrogens.

Xenoestrogens convert to estrogen. Also, remember that excess estrogen will hamper the ability of thyroid hormone to get into the cells. BPA, pesticides, herbicides, nail polish remover and drycleaning materials are all xenoestrogens. Cattle and poultry are fed with estrogen-like hormones. Be on the lookout for any possible exposures and avoid them; i.e., do not microwave plastics.

When it comes to soy and phytoestrogens, keep in mind that they are 1/60th the strength of estrogen. Your focus should be on avoiding xenoestrogens.

An option to increase progesterone is the use of sublingual plant based progesterone. A company named Apex offers a product called Progestaid which contains nutritional compounds to promote healthy progesterone production.

It is less often the case that estrogen needs to be raised. However, sublingual DHEA can convert to estrogen and increase the estrogen levels. Insulin resistance must be addressed. There are plant-based bio-identical forms of estrogen including a prescription product called Triest/Biest. Herbal approaches include black cohosh, dong quai and shepherd's purse.

Synthetic Hormones

All studies showing ill effects of HRT hormone replacement were done using **synthetic** hormones; e.g., Provera/ Premarin, not bio-identical. Synthetic hormones are toxic to the body while bio-identicals are not.

The Women's Health Initiative and other studies showed that taking synthetic estrogen and progesterone increased the risk of heart disease and cancer. In fact, the study was terminated early as women began to develop cancer and heart disease.

If needed, use **bio-identical** hormones.

Hypothyroid Autoimmune Diet (Phase 1)

I f you have Hashimoto's and you are disciplined and motivated, begin with the autoimmune diet for 4-12 weeks. If you have addictions to food or you feel it would be impossible to follow the autoimmune diet, then start by eliminating gluten, dairy and soy. As you develop better eating habits, you can make further eliminations. There are advanced food sensitivity tests available which will be discussed in later chapters that can pinpoint exactly which foods you should eliminate.

In a nutshell, the autoimmune diet is free of: grains, dairy, eggs, all sweeteners, nightshades (potatoes, tomatoes, peppers, eggplant) and processed foods. What is left is a diet that focuses on plenty of vegetables, cultured vegetables (such as sauerkraut) and healthy meats and fats. You should eat regularly enough to avoid drops in blood sugar and drink plenty of filtered or spring water.

Because the diet is rather stringent, grabbing a quick meal while you're out or conjuring a meal from an empty fridge is tricky. The most important strategy for success is planning and preparation. You have to be one step ahead of yourself when it comes to future meals. Some essentials of the diet include:

a) Grass fed meats

The ideal types of meat on the diet are pastured meats raised on small farms. The animals are free from hormones, antibiotics, and GMO feeds. Because grass-fed meats have become so popular, you may be able to find them on small farms in your area or at health food stores. US Wellness Meats is an online source that can ship a wide variety of frozen pastured meats to your home.

b) Coconut Oil

Coconut oil is a staple diet, taking the place of butter for many cooking needs (unless you are sensitive to it, which some people are). Thankfully, coconut oil is becoming more commonplace on the shelves of health food stores and even at Costco. Tropical Traditions was one of the first to offer coconut oil for sale online and continues to offer premium oils.

c) Cultured Foods

Consuming cultured foods and drinks helps restore a healthy balance of gut flora. To the newcomer, fermenting, culturing, and making kefir can seem foreign and even risky.

Cultures for Health provides plenty of easy how-to articles and videos, as well as starter cultures.

I recommend following the autoimmune diet listed below for a period of 4-12 weeks. If you have Hashimoto's or an autoimmune disease, you should commit to at least 12 weeks. After the initial 4-12 period, move to the mainte-nance diet I have listed below.

So, to recap, start with the Autoimmune Diet (Phase 1) for weeks 4-12.

Foods to Eat

a) Most organic vegetables: including anise, artichoke, asparagus, beets, bok choy, broccoli, cabbage, carrot, cauliflower, celery, chives, cucumber, garlic, kale, kohlrabi, leeks, lettuce, mustard greens, onions, parsley, radish, rhubarb, shallots, spinach, squash, sweet potatoes, water chestnuts, watercress, yams, zucchini

b) Fermented Foods: including kimchi, kombucha tea, pickled ginger, sauerkraut, unsweetened coconut yogurt

c) Meats: including beef, chicken, fish, lamb, turkey. Fish should be ocean caught with a low-mercury content. Swordfish, most tuna, and king mackerel are very high in mercury. Select hormone-free and antibiotic-free chicken, turkey, lamb and beef that is grass-fed, hormone free, and antibiotic-free.

d) Low Glycemic Organic Fruits: including apples, apricots, avocados, berries, cherries, grapefruit, grapes, lemons, oranges, peaches, pears, plums.

e) Coconut: including coconut butter, coconut cream, coconut milk, coconut oil, unsweetened coconut flakes, unsweetened coconut yogurt.

f) Noodles: brown shirataki yam noodles (sold in Asian grocery stores).

g) Herbs and Spices: including basil, black pepper, cilantro, coriander, cumin, garlic, ginger, lemongrass, mint, oregano, parsley, rosemary, sage, sea salt, thyme.

h) Other: apple cider vinegar, herbal teas, olive oil, olives.

Foods to Avoid:

a) Sugars: including agave, candy, chocolate, corn syrup, fructose, high fructose corn syrup, honey, maple syrup, molasses, and sucrose.

b) High Glycemic Fruits: including bananas, canned fruits, dried fruits, mango, pineapple, raisins, and watermelon.

c) Grains: including amaranth, barley, buckwheat, bulgur, corn, couscous, kamut, millet, oats, quinoa, rice, rye, spelt, wheat, wheat germ.

d) Nuts and Seeds: including almonds, peanuts, sunflower seeds, sesame seeds.

e) Gluten-Containing Compounds: including barbecue sauce, binders, bouillon, brewer's yeast, cold cuts, condiments, emulsifiers, fillers, gum, hot dogs, hydrolyzed plant and vegetable protein, ketchup, soy sauce, lunch meats, malt and malt flavoring, malt vinegar, matzo, modified food starch, monosodium glutamate (MSG), nondairy creamer, processed salad dressings, seitan, some spice mixtures, stabilizers, teriyaki sauce, textured vegetable protein.

f) Dairy Products and Eggs: including butter, cheeses, cow milk, creams, frozen desserts, goat milk, margarine, mayonnaise, sheep milk, whey, yogurt (except coconut).

g) Soy: including edamame, miso, soy milk, soy protein, soy sauce, tempeh, and tofu.

h) Fungi: edible fungi and mushrooms.

i) Alcohol: all alcohol.

j) Beans and Legumes: including black beans, lentils, peanuts, peas, pinto beans and soybeans.

k) Nightshades: including eggplant, paprika, peppers, potatoes, Tabasco sauce, tomatillos and tomatoes.

l) Other: canned foods, coffee and processed foods.

Phase 1 of the Autoimmune Diet is the most challenging part of getting better and I will share with you how we help patients through this stage. One of the suggestions I have for my patients is to make smoothies. Get yourself a Vitamix or Ninja and use the recipe guide I have outlined below. Be creative and make something you enjoy. The convenience and ease will help you through the 4-12 week period.

Smoothie Recipe

Unsweetened Coconut Milk

Spinach or kale (or any green leafy vegetables) or any combination of vegetables

Half or whole avocado (cut the avocado in half, remove seed and squeeze or scoop the contents

Frozen or fresh fruit* (this can be any that you prefer)

*If you use fresh fruit, use ice cubes to give it a smoothie feel

I also use one scoop of pea protein (10-15 grams)

After the initial 4-12 week period, you can begin to add foods back. This is where lab testing is useful as tests can identify what you are sensitive to and may allow you to have a broader diet than without testing. Reintroduction is a method that we previously used prior to testing. The problem with reintroduction is that in the absence of symptoms you still could have sensitivities. For example, you would add eggs back first for 3 days. If you had no symptoms, we would assume that would be OK. I have outlined a Maintenance Diet below which you could follow after completion of the Autoimmune Diet.

Helpful tips

Little snacks for on-the-go:

- Sliced deli meat (Applegate brand)
- Pea Protein shake (http://www.sunwarrior.com). Mix with water, coconut milk or coconut water.
- Cucumbers with olive oil, lemon salt and pepper dressing
- Dill pickles
- Apple, peach, nectarine, cherries
- Coconut yogurt
- Cucumbers and guacamole
- Epic Protein Bar (www.epicbar.com)
- Coconut yogurt (plain) with a half scoop of chocolate protein powder and mix well.
- A greens juice (kale, broccoli, cucumber, lemon, ginger, green apple and beets)
- Tuna salad with celery sticks and cucumber (canned tuna with lemon, salt, pepper, olives, onion, and celery) - be creative! Be sure to buy tuna that is free of metals. You may want to look at wild salmon in a bag.
- Lettuce wraps (sliced deli meat, avocado wrapped up in butter lettuce and dipped in olive oil and vinegar dressing)

Breakfast ideas:

- Chicken/Turkey sausage (Applegate is a great brand)
- You can eat a half grapefruit or some berries, apple, etc. at breakfast

- Salmon/lox for breakfast; good with some capers or red onion

- Some sweet potato hash with onions, some cinnamon sautéed with coconut oil. Can be made in a big batch ahead of time and reheated

- A piece of turkey in a muffin pan; break an egg (when eggs are added back in) into it or scramble the egg and pour in; bake in an oven at 350 for about 10 or 16 minutes until done. Top with avocado, some dairy-free; e.g. Daiya cheese and some sea salt and cracked pepper

Here are some resources that will also help:

- www.gfreelife.com

- www.ceceliasmarketplace.com – she has a book called the *Gluten Free, Casein Free and a Soy-Free Shopping Guide*

- www.marksdailyapple.com – Primal living/Caveman food plans

- www.whfoods.com – World's Healthiest Foods

- www.glutenfreechecklist.com

- www.facebook.com/JustEatingRealFood

- www.paleomom.com Autoimmune diets

Maintenance Diet (Phase 2)

When you have completed Phase 1 of the autoimmune diet, you can proceed to the Maintenance Diet (Phase 2).

It's important to shop for quality foods at butcher's shops, farmers markets, fish markets and natural food stores. The worst foods to cheat with are going to be gluten (wheat, barley, rye, spelt), dairy and soy proteins.

Basic Guidelines:

1. Eat 4-6 small meals per day.
2. Make sure you eat within 1 hour of rising in the morning.
3. Always have some fat when you eat a fruit. For example, an apple plus a handful of almonds
4. Eat twice as many vegetables as fruit over the course of the day. Raw vegetables are best if you want to lose weight.
5. Remember that eating this way will be new and sometimes a challenge to achieve.
6. Preparing single servings of food that can be frozen will save you from having to cook meals when life gets busy.
7. Prepare large batches of staples like spaghetti sauce and soups for freezing in single serve containers. If you must reheat food in the microwave, transfer the food to a glass container. Plastic releases harmful chemicals into your food when heated in a microwave.

Foods Specific Guidelines:

Meats: (from best to worst): Fish, Wild Game (venison, bison), Chicken, Beef, Turkey, Pork. Vary the other meats in frequency. Cured meats like ham, bacon and sausage can be eaten but not as an everyday staple. "Al Fresco" is a great chicken sausage that is gluten free, dairy free, nitrate free and available at local grocers. Organic, grass fed, free range is best. If it is wrapped in plastic or packaged, you probably don't want to eat it.

Seafood: 4-5 servings of fish a week is recommended. Avoid farm-raised fish. Smoked salmon is acceptable.

Vegetables: Fresh veggies are best. Multiple colors are even better. Eat at least a couple of servings of raw veggies per day. This is where you will get most of your really good minerals and vitamins. Focus on what is in season. Pass on veggies in cans. Kale is a versatile lettuce that works well in salads, sautés and soups and is your best choice for nutrition. Sweet potatoes are okay but skip the white potatoes. Spaghetti squash is a staple for us. Always keep spaghetti sauce available for a quick meal. Add different meats each time for variety.

Grains: Avoid rice but try quinoa. It is a grain with a nutty flavor and works well as a substitute for rice and potatoes.

Salads: Choose dark green leafy lettuces like kale, spinach or spring mix. Avoid iceberg altogether. Use many different vegetables in your salads and always top with some sort of protein. Grilled chicken, fish, beef, shrimp are some of our favorites. Nuts and fruit are great in salads. Avoid bottled salad dressings. Choose vinegar and oil or seasonings to spice up your salad. Juice from a half lemon or orange also makes a great dressing.

All Fruits: 2-3 servings per day. Keep in mind this is a sugar source and sugar addicts can easily eat too much fruit. Frozen berries are OK, in small amounts. Diabetics should be very careful here. Wash all fruit prior to eating it.

Eggs: Farm fresh, no egg substitutes. Yolks ARE good for you. Eat them.

Broth: For soups. Read the labels and make sure there is not gluten or other thickening agents. Choose low sodium brands or use the water from blanching vegetables and cooking meats as your broth.

Nuts: Raw nuts are best but roasted are also okay. Avoid nuts that are salted and covered in honey. Choose a variety but watch the amount if you wish to lose weight. A serving of nuts should be the equivalent of 8 almonds.

Drinks: Water with lemon is going to be the drink of choice. Have a 32 fluid ounce bottle filled in the morning and drink it by lunch. Repeat in the afternoon. Seltzer water and herbal tea is OK also. Coffee and alcohol are no-no's. Almond milk (unsweetened if you are diabetic) and coconut milk. If you need a sweetener, try Stevia.

Cooking Oils: Sauté with olive oil. If you need to use higher temps, use Coconut Oil. If I let you eat dairy, then butter is ok, not margarine. Canola oil, vegetable oil, corn oil and soybean oils are BAD.

Spices: All are OK. Use sea salt. Keep salt to under 1,500 mg. if blood pressure is an issue.

Desserts: Coconut ice cream is a special treat and should be savored. Baking fruit like apples and peaches are fabulous alternatives to processed desserts. Use spices to add flavor.

Snacks: Hummus with carrot and celery sticks is a favorite. You can purchase pre- made brands or make your own with garbanzo, black or Northern white beans. Organic almond or cashew butter is a better choice than peanut butter but as long as it is organic and natural, peanut butter is fine. No processed brands like Skippy or Jif. Whole food snack bars like Macro or Kind may be eaten as a snack, ½ bar at a time, no more than one bar per day.

Starches, carbohydrates and gluten free foods:
Rice, tapioca, sweet potato, quinoa, buckwheat, and millet are gluten-free. Bob's Red Mill also makes a gluten-free oatmeal. I would suggest staying away from wheat products (gluten). As I mentioned, food testing from Cyrex or ELISA ACT can help you determine if you have any sensitivities to these foods. Following a gluten-free diet is good. However, I have many patients that are sensitive to certain gluten-free foods. If you have an autoimmune condition, get tested. Without testing, it's best to stay away from these foods.

Carbohydrate Addiction

Scientists may have confirmed what millions of us could have already told you: One cookie is too many and 20 are not enough. Many people have found they can go along comfortably on a diet free of sweets, pastries, and desserts until they have that one bite. Then—zing!—the addiction sets in and you feel like you might die if you don't eat more. Turns out you're not weak or gluttonous. It's just your brain responding to the highly pleasurable and stimulating effect of cookies, cake, chips, and candy as if they were powerful drugs (which, really, they are). It's no mystery why they're also referred to as comfort foods.

These processed carbohydrates appeal to the same parts of the brain involved in substance abuse and addiction, as anyone with a carb addiction can tell you. A major player in addiction is the neurotransmitter dopamine, which gives us the feeling of reward and pleasure associated with activities that can be addictive. For instance, drug use, smoking and gambling all release dopamine. In rat studies, rats given the option of pressing a lever that stimulates dopamine's pleasurable effects or a lever for food chose the dopamine to their death.

In the recent study, researchers gave two groups of overweight men a milkshake. One group's milkshake was higher on the glycemic index than the other group. This means it was sweeter and more processed, causing blood sugar to rise more quickly and then crash. Four hours later, researchers scanned the brains of both groups using an MRI. The men receiving the high-glycemic milkshake felt excessively hungry and scans revealed intense activation in the area of the brain involved in addiction. These brain changes can trigger overeating.

Avoid high-glycemic foods

Not triggering the pleasure centers of your brain with food is one of your most powerful allies in healthier eating and weight loss. Eating a whole foods diet that is satiating and prevents hunger is key to curbing cravings and taming carb addiction. This means including healthy proteins and fats to stabilize your blood sugar and sustain your energy, as well as plenty of vegetables for the fiber, which also helps keep your energy on an even keel.

The glycemic index measures how quickly foods become glucose after you eat them. The glycemic load factors in the amount of the carbohydrate eaten. So, although a piece of candy has a high glycemic index, the glycemic load might be small if you eat a very small piece.

High-glycemic foods that can trigger carb addiction include:

- White potato
- White rice
- White bread, bagels, muffins, rolls, etc.
- Pastries, cake, cookies, etc.
- Breakfast cereal
- Popcorn

- Dried fruit
- Ripe banana
- Soft drinks
- Fruit juice
- Pizza
- Candy bars

GMO's

Scientific studies are showing that genetically engineered foods, or genetically modified organisms (GMOs), can damage the organs of the body, including the liver, kidneys and brain. Researchers also found significant changes that affected weight gain, eating behaviors, and immune function.

You won't get sick from one meal containing GM corn or soy (just as you won't get sick from one pack, or even 10 packs, of cigarettes) but most people have far greater exposure.

About 90% of America's corn, cotton, soy, canola and sugar beet crops are genetically engineered. You will find GMOs in fresh produce and processed foods and in such animal products as milk, meat and eggs because of GM animal feed.

The GMO industry claims its crops are safe, but even before Monsanto, the international agricultural biotechnology corporation, was allowed to plant its first commercial crop in 1996, Food and Drug Administration scientists were calling for more research. They predicted that engineered foods would contain rogue proteins that could be toxic and cause allergies, nutritional deficiencies and other diseases. Their calls for better testing were ignored.

GMO foods and crops are closely regulated in Europe. According to the European Commission, the rules are in place "to protect human and animal health through stringent safety assessment of GM food and feed before it can be sold" and "to ensure clear labeling that responds to the concerns of consumers and enables them to make informed choices."

Why is the U.S. policy so different? Food and agricultural companies spent millions to defeat California's proposition demanding better food labeling, a move that thrust GMOs into the spotlight. Many weren't aware about the GMOs in their foods until that battle.

Then, the Farmer's Assurance Provision (a/k/a the Monsanto Protection Act) was tacked onto a U.S. spending bill in March, 2014. It actually requires that the Dept. of Agriculture ignore a Court Order and allow the planting of new genetically engineered crops while the agency conducts further review.

The best way to avoid GMOs is to buy organic foods or foods with the Non-GMO Project seal. When buying conventional foods, avoid those with corn, soy, canola, cottonseed and "sugar"

(but not "cane sugar") as ingredients! You can also download a shopping guide at (NonGmoShoppingGuide. com) to help you steer clear of GMOs.

How safe are GMOs?

More often than not, unless the research is tainted by industry ties, studies into the effects of genetically engineered foods demonstrate that it is anything but safe. This isn't so surprising when you consider that simple logic will tell you it's probably not wise to consume a plant designed to produce its own pesticide, for example.

So-called "Bt corn" is equipped with a gene from the soil bacteria Bacillus thuringiensis (Bt), which produces Bt-toxin—a pesticide that breaks open the stomach of certain insects and kills them. This pesticide-producing corn entered the food supply in the late 1990's, and over the past decade, the horror stories have started piling up.

Monsanto and the U.S. Environmental Protection Agency (EPA) swore that the toxin would only affect insects munching on the crop. The Bt-toxin, they claimed, would be completely destroyed in the human digestive system and would not impact animals and humans. The biotech companies have doggedly insisted that Bt-toxin doesn't bind or interact with the intestinal walls of mammals, and therefore humans. The research proves all such claims false.

Prior findings have already shown that Bt corn is anything but innocuous to the human system. Just last year, doctors at Sherbrooke University Hospital in Quebec found Bt-toxin in the blood of:

- 93 percent of pregnant women tested
- 80 percent of these women's umbilical blood in their babies, and
- 67 percent of non-pregnant women

Bt-toxin breaks open the stomach of insects. Could it similarly be damaging the integrity of your digestive tract? If Bt-toxins can damage the intestinal walls of newborns and young children, the passage of undigested foods and toxins into the blood from the digestive tract could be devastating to their future health. Scientists speculate that it may lead to autoimmune diseases and food allergies. Furthermore, since the blood-brain barrier is not developed in newborns, toxins may enter the brain causing serious cognitive problems. Some healthcare practitioners and scientists are convinced that this is one mechanism for autism.

If Bt genes are colonizing the bacteria living in the digestive tract of North Americans, we might expect to see an increase in gastrointestinal problems, autoimmune diseases, food allergies, and childhood learning disorders since the advent of Bt crops in 1996 and that is

exactly what's being reported. For example, between 1997 and 2002, the number of hospitalizations related to allergic reactions to food increased by a whopping 265 percent. One out of 17 children now has some form of food allergy and allergy rates are rising.

So-called "Roundup Ready" crops are another type of genetically engineered crops. While Bt crops contain a gene that produces a pesticide inside the plant itself, Roundup Ready crops are designed to withstand otherwise lethal topical doses of glyphosate, a broad spectrum herbicide, and the active ingredient in Monsanto's herbicide Roundup as well as hundreds of other products.

This way, the crop survives while theoretically all weeds are eliminated from the field ... that is 'theoretically' because the overuse of the herbicide has led to the rapid development of glyphosate-resistant superweeds. It is estimated that more than 130 types of weeds spanning 40 U.S. states are now herbicide-resistant and the superweeds are showing no signs of stopping.

Roundup Ready crops have also been linked to serious health problems—particularly relating to fertility and birth defects—as has glyphosate itself.

Top 10 Worst GMO Foods that you should Avoid Eating

a) Corn – Corn is one of the most prominent GMO foods. Avoiding corn is a no-brainer. If you've watched any food documentary, you know corn is highly modified. Monsanto's GMO corn has been tied to many health issues, including weight gain and organ disruption.

b) Soy - found in tofu, vegetarian products, soybean oil, soy flour, and numerous other products. Soy is also modified to resist herbicides. As of now, biotech giant Monsanto still has a tight grasp on the soybean market, with approximately 90 percent of soy being genetically engineered to resist Monsanto's herbicide, Roundup.

c) Sugar - Genetically-modified sugar beets were introduced to the U.S. market in 2009. Like others, they've been modified by Monsanto to resist herbicides.

d) Aspartame is a toxic additive used in numerous food products and should be avoided for numerous reasons, including the fact that it is created with genetically modified bacteria.

e) Papayas – GMO papayas have been grown in Hawaii for consumption since 1999. Although they can't be sold to countries in the European Union, they are welcomed with open arms in the U.S. and Canada.

f) Canola is one of the most chemically altered foods in the U.S. diet. Canola oil is obtained from rapeseed through a series of chemical actions.

g) Cotton - Found in cotton oil, cotton originating in India and China in particular has serious risks.

h) Dairy - Your dairy products may contain growth hormones, since as many as one-fifth of all dairy cows in America are pumped full of these hormones. In fact, Monsanto's health-hazardous rBGH has been banned in 27 countries but is still in most US cows. If you must drink milk, buy organic.

i) Zucchini and Yellow Squash - these two squash varieties are modified to resist viruses.

CHAPTER 4:
BLOOD TESTING AND VALUES

have listed some blood tests which include functional ranges (optimal ranges). This is the range you want for optimal function and ideal health. Some of the ranges might be narrower than what is listed on your lab tests (the 'reference range'). However, it is a way to pick up shifts in health that might lead to diseases - allowing us to catch a problem before it manifests as a disease. I have listed many of the tests that I use. So, to be clear, the ranges I include below are **functional ranges** for optimal health. The labs use broader reference ranges to identify the disease.

If you are outside of the lab's reference range, you should consult with a Medical Doctor.

Below is a complete list of thyroid tests along with a description:

1. TSH (1.8-3.0) – TSH is secreted by the pituitary gland. If the thyroid is not making enough thyroid hormone, the pituitary will pump extra TSH (thyroid stimulating hormone) to attempt to increase production. This is one of the tests commonly looked at by the conventional health care model and is primarily used to evaluate the need for and effectiveness of thyroid hormone replacement.

   A high TSH is indicative of hypothyroidism (low thyroid production).

A low TSH is indicative of hyperthyroidism (low meaning below 0.5) – which may be Graves's disease. If so, you would also see T4 and T3 levels high. In such a case, an antibody test for Graves is needed (TSI antibody).

A TSH between 0.5 and 1.8 without being on medication is indicative of a problem with the pituitary. If a patient is on medication and is having heart palpitations, then the patient might be overmedicated.

The TSH does not consider thyroid metabolism, autoimmune disease or thyroid pituitary feedback loops. Many patients have a normal TSH and feel horrible. TSH alone will not to get to the cause of the problem.

2. Total T4 (6—12 mcg./dl.)- T4 is produced by the thyroid gland and total T4 is a measure of T4 that is bound by proteins and unbound by proteins. This number does not tell us how active T4 is. T3 uptake is used to indicate how much hormone is entering the cell.

    Low- would lead us to consider hypothyroidism

    High- would lead us to consider hyperthyroidism

3. Total T3 (100-190 ng./dl.) - T3 is the most active thyroid hormone and is produced mainly from the conversion of T4 to T3 in the body. The thyroid gland produces 93% T4 and 7% T3.

    Low- would lead us to consider hypothyroidism

    High- would lead us to consider hyperthyroidism

4. Free T4 (1.0-1.5 ng./dl.) - Measures T4 that is not bound by protein and is more available for tissue receptors. Hereditary thyroid resistance can cause increased Free T4.

    Low- would lead us to consider hypothyroidism

    High- would lead us to consider hyperthyroidism

5. Free T3 (3.0-4.0 pg./ml.)- Measures T3 that is not bound by protein and is most available to the thyroid receptor sites.

   Low- would lead us to consider hypothyroidism

   High- would lead us to consider hyperthyroidism

6. T3 Uptake (28-35%) - Measures the amount of open receptor sites for T3. A low value means there are not many sites available. A high value means that there are plenty of open sites available. High levels of testosterone can decrease the number of sites and high levels of estrogen can increase the number of sites. This test is an indirect way to determine if hormones are affecting thyroid function.

   Low- would lead us to consider hypothyroidism

   High- would lead us to consider hyperthyroidism

7. Reverse T3 (90-350 pg./ml.) – Is produced in the liver. The liver will convert T4 to T3 or reverse T3. You should have a healthy balance. Some schools of thought suggest using a ratio of reverse T3 to Total T3. Divide Total T3 by Reverse T3. That value should be 10 or greater for healthy thyroid function.

8. Thyroid Binding Globulin (18-27 ug./dl.) (TBG) – measures the amount of protein available to transport thyroid hormone to the cells. Elevated testosterone or estrogen levels can influence the amount of TBG available producing hypothyroid symptoms.

9. Thyroid Antibodies - If you have any symptoms of thyroid dysfunction, it is wise to screen for autoimmune disease or activity. I have consulted with patients that had completely normal thyroid lab values and tested positive for antibodies against the thyroid. This test will tell you if your immune system is attacking the thyroid (most commonly known as Hashimoto's disease). There are two tests to check: TPOab Thyroid Peroxidase and Thyroglobulin ab TGBab (for Hashimoto's). TSIab

47

thyroid stimulating immunoglobulin antibody is used to test for Grave's Disease (hyperthyroid).

Normal result: no antibodies produced.

The above tests are needed to appropriately evaluate thyroid function. The goal would be to achieve normal functional values. Below I have supplied a list of other blood tests and values that I use in evaluating patients. These tests give me a complete starting point in evaluating the health status of a patient.

Test	Functional Range	Result	High/Low	Weakness/Possibilities
GLUCOSE	85 – 100 mg/dL		Normal High Low	The body's chief source of energy. It affects all organs, systems and tissues. High levels of blood sugar are inflam-matory. This is a precursor to heart disease. • Hyperglycemic tendency toward diabetes, lack of exercise, low thiamine, questionable diet. • Hypoglycemia, hypothyroidism, excessive insulin output, protein malnutrition.
URIC ACID	Male: 3.7 – 6.0 mg/dL Female: 3.2 – 5.5 mg/dL		Normal High Low	End product of protein utilization. Meat, wine (especially liver, kidneys), shellfish and beans are high in uric acid. • Gout, arteriosclerosis., rheumatoid arthritis, Kidney problems • Low B12, incomplete protein digestion, acidic pH, low in zinc and niacin.; copper deficiency

Test	Functional Range	Result	High/Low	Weakness/Possibilities
BUN	13 – 18 mg/dL		Normal High Low	Reveals the degree of toxicity of protein to the kidneys. Too much urea production by liver or not cleared by kidneys • Renal problems, dehydration, hypochlo-rydria (lack of stomach acid), high protein diet, stress, liver, thyroid, parathyroid imbalance, kidney obstruction (e.g., stones), low Vitamin A, C and/or E, potassium, abnormal blood loss • Pregnancy, liver dysfunction, low protein or protein malnu-trition, heavy smoking, tendency toward diabetes.
CREATININE	0.7 – 1.1 mg/dL		Normal High Low	Relates to muscle activity and renal functioning. Kidneys clear creatinine. • Dehydration, kidney problems, prostate enlargement indicates muscle breakdown to supply protein, high ingestion of meats, supplementation of creatine can cause high levels (It does not mean creatine is bad. Kidneys are just doing their job); check BUN also and liver AST and ALT • Pregnancy, bone growth, overstress to kidney (heavy coffee, tea, alcohol), too much Vitamin C compulsive exercise.

Test	Functional Range	Result	High/Low	Weakness/Possibilities
SODIUM Electrolyte formula	135 – 140 mmol/L 9-18 optimal		Normal High Low	Essential to acid-base balance and intra/extra-cellular fluid exchanges for normal body water distribution. • Renal problems, water softeners, high sodium-salt diet, low water intake, relates to toxins, headaches, weak back muscles, low potassium levels, fluid imbalance and lack of physical activity. High adrenal function • Low adrenal function, low salt diet, lack of trace minerals, loss of fluids & loss of sodium in diarrhea or vomit. (Sodium) – (CL + CO2) = 9-18 optimal
POTASSIUM	4.0 – 4.5 mmol/L		Normal High Low	Essential to heart & kidney function and the mainte-nance of pH of both blood & urine. It maintains regular heart rate and muscle force, thus helps to prevent heart and general muscle fatigue. • Low adrenal, dehydration, low kidney function, overuse of potassium supplements, relates to congestive heart failure and renal failure, low vitamin E, insufficient exercise and deep breathing • Tissue destruction, high adrenal, renal problems, diabetes, tendency toward weak heart, alcohol related, folic acid deficiency, low fluid intake, low potassium intake, low vegetable and fruit intake; diuretics

Test	Functional Range	Result	High/Low	Weakness/Possibilities
CHLORIDE (CL)	100 – 106 mmol/L		Normal High Low	Indicates kidney, bladder, and bowel function. Essential for electrolyte balance and pH maintenance. • High adrenal, excess salt, renal dysfunction, high salt intake, severe dehydration, could relate to bowel dysfunction, insufficient green vegetables, liver malfunction, magnesium deficiency • Low adrenal, low renal function, B12 deficiency, susceptible to infections, tendency toward colitis, bladder dysfunction.
CARBON DIOXIDE (CO2)	25 -30 mmol/L		Normal High Low	Bicarbonate is a vital component of controlling the pH of the body. Regulated by the kidneys. • Alkalosis most commonly seen with lung disease or emphysema • Acidosis can result in serious illness or kidney disease
ANION GAP	7 – 12 mmol/L		Normal High Low	Helps differentiate the causes of metabolic acidosis. • Low thiamine (B1), metabolic acidosis, kidneys • Very rare

Test	Functional Range	Result	High/Low	Weakness/Possibilities
CALCIUM	9.2 – 10.1 mg/dL9.7		Normal High Low	The majority of calcium is stored in the bone (98-99%). This is not a measure of stored calcium. The body uses the stored calcium to draw into circulation which is measured here. Calcium in the blood is used for cardiac regularity, muscle relaxation & contraction, blood clotting, transmission of nerve impulses. • Parathyroid hyper-function, thyroid hypo-function, excess Vitamin D use, bone disorders, possibility of calcium not being absorbed, lack of exercise or possible thyroid/parathyroid gland malfunction. • Pregnancy, osteo-porosis, low thyroid/parathyroid gland malfunction. Malnutrition, Vitamin D deficiency
PHOSPHORUS	3.5 – 4.0 mg/dL		Normal High Low	Critical constituent of all the body's tissues. Majority is stored in bone. Inversely related to calcium • Parathyroid hypo. function, bone fracture, kids' bone growth, renal dysfunction • Parathyroid hyper function, hypoch-lorhydria (lack of stomach acid), low protein, blood sugar problems, Vitamin D deficiency

Test	Functional Range	Result	High/Low	Weakness/Possibilities
MAGNESIUM	2.0 – 2.5 mg/dL		Normal High Low	Critical to smooth muscle function, including heart, gastrointestinal tract and uterus; helps regulate acid-alkaline (base) balance in the body. Aids in absorption and metabolism of minerals such as calcium, phosphorus, sodium, and potassium; also utilization of Vitamin B complex, C and E. Regulates body temperature. If the magnesium is found intra-cellularly, this is not the best method for assessing magnesium. *Run the red blood cell magnesium for more accurate assessment of magnesium* • Kidney dysfunction, low thyroid, infection • Supplement use, malnutrition, alcoholism, and excessive use of diuretics.
TOTAL PROTEIN	6.9 – 7.4 G/dL		Normal High Low	Screen for digestive problems, dehydration. • Need HCl, amino acids and protein (indicates incomplete assimilation or non-use of protein) dehydration or loss of fluid. • Need HCl, amino acids, protein (incomplete protein digestion), poor nutrition, liver dysfunction.

Test	Functional Range	Result	High/Low	Weakness/Possibilities
ALBUMIN	4.0 – 5.0 G/dL		Normal High Low	A major protein in the blood that transports hormones and drugs. Dehydration, protein gram overload or absorption, hypothyroidism. • Starvation/malnu- trition, edema, liver/ kidney problems, Vitamin C deficiency, hyperthyroidism • Heavy aspirin use, liver, bile, decreased immune function
GLOBULIN	– 2.8 G/dL		Normal High Low	Essential to the antibody-antigen response; needed to fight infections; important in blood clotting. Valuable in assessing degenerative and infec- tious processes. • Hypochlorhydria (lack of stomach acid), allergy, a sign of arthritis • Digestive dysfunction, immune system deficiency, liver disease, inflammation, infection related
A/G RATIO	1.5 – 2.0 Units		Normal High Low	Relates to the body's defense mechanism; associated with the liver. • Usually due to dehydration; not enough water before the test • Liver dysfunction, Immune system activation.

Test	Functional Range	Result	High/Low	Weakness/Possibilities
TOTAL BILIRUBIN	0.2 – 1.2 mg/dL		Normal High Low	Bilirubin is the end product of hemoglobin breakdown from red blood cells in the spleen and bone marrow. It is transported to the liver and then the gallbladder where it is eventually excreted. Two types: direct and indirect. High levels of indirect are usually associated with increased cell destruction. High levels of direct are associated with liver or gallbladder problems. • Fat malabsorption & increased risk of cardiovascular disease, possible lymphatic problems, Vitamin C deficiency; potential liver disease or jaundice. Spleen Dysfunction • Spleen insufficiency, iron deficiency, anemia, Vitamins B-12 and C and copper deficiency
ALK. PHOSPHATASE	70 – 90 U/L		Normal High Low	Indicates how the liver is utilizing protein and fats, and pH balance (an enzyme found essentially in bone & liver) • Bone growth, liver dysfunction, gastric inflammation, tendency towards arthritis, insufficient calcium/phosphorus could relate to certain medications, bile duct obstruction, or alcohol related. • Protein malnutrition, Vitamin C, folic acid and zinc deficiency; possible hypoglycemia

Test	Functional Range	Result	High/Low	Weakness/Possibilities
LDH	140 – 180 U/L		Normal High Low	LDH is a catalyst for the conversion of pyruvic acid to lactic acid during cellular energy production • Liver problems, cardiac stress, diabetic tendency, strenuous exercise, alcohol related, present in myocardial infarction & pulmonary conditions • Reactive hypogly-cemia, possible edema and fatigue.
AST (SGOT)	10 – 26 U/L		Normal High Low	Relates to liver enzyme activity, kidney & skeletal muscle • Liver complications, heart or muscle problems • Low B6 levels and magnesium deficiency
ALT (SGPT)	10 – 26 U/L		Normal High Low	An enzyme associated with the liver, heart and skeletal muscle. • Liver dysfunction, alcohol and drug related, Vitamins A and C deficiency • Low B6 levels, alcohol
GGTP	10 – 26 U/L		Normal High Low	An excellent indicator of liver damage or biliary obstruction of bile ducts outside the liver • Alcoholism, bile obstruction, viral hepatitis • Low B6 levels and copper, hypothyroid, low magnesium

Test	Functional Range	Result	High/Low	Weakness/ Possibilities
IRON SERUM	85 – 130 mcg/dL		Normal High Low	Critical to red blood cells' ability to carry oxygen & remove carbon dioxide; helps to remove toxin residue from cells. • Hemochromatosis is a hereditary disorder (excess absorption of iron), liver problems. Increase iron intake (supplements), iron cookware, drinking water • Iron deficiency, internal or external bleeding.
FERRITIN	Male: 33—236 Female: 10—122 Post menopausal: 33- 263		Normal High Low	The most sensitive test to detect iron deficiency. Main storage form of iron in the body • Hemochromatosis (excess absorption of iron), inflammation, excess iron consumption • Iron- deficiency anemia
TIBC	250-350 ul/dl		Normal High Low	Total iron binding capacity. Measures the blood's capacity to bind iron • Iron deficiency • Hemochromatosis (excess absorption of iron)

Test	Functional Range	Result	High/Low	Weakness/ Possibilities
HEMOGLOBIN A1C	4.8--5.6 5.7—6.4 >6.4		Normal High Higher	Measures blood glucose that has attached itself to protein (albumin). This test more accurately measures glucose levels over the two-three weeks prior to the blood test • Increased risk for diabetes • Diabetes
CHOLESTEROL	150 – 200 mg/dL		Normal High Low	Cholesterol is found in every cell of the body. Used to make hormones, enzymes, antibodies & all cells. It is manufactured in the liver. Cannot function without it. • Hypothyroidism, early stage of diabetes, low thiamine, excessive dietary fats (hydrogenated oils), lack of Vitamins A, C, D, E, stress, • smoking, insuffiient exercise • Hyperthyroidism, protein malnutrition, alcoholism, carbs, cholesterol medication. It is not wise to have levels below 150.

Test	Functional Range	Result	High/Low	Weakness/ Possibilities
Triglycerides/ HDL Ratio* TRIGLY- CERIDES	Divide ratio 75 – 100 mg/dL	2	High Normal High Low	Increased risk of heart disease - goal is 2. For example, Triglycerides 100/HDL 50 = 2. The goal is a ratio of 2, an excellent marker for heart disease. Are major building blocks of very low density lipoproteins (VLDL) and play an important role in metabolism as energy sources and trans- porters of dietary fat • Blood sugar problems, sugar & saturated fat eaters, stress related, increased risk of heart and small vessel diseases, poor exercise habits • Autoimmune disease, nerves & stress related, protein malnu- trition, excessive use of bran & niacin, low unsatu- rated fatty acids
HDL "GOOD" CHOLESTEROL	>55 mg/dl--- <80 mg/dl		Normal High Low	The "good" choles- terol; it carries choles- terol away from your arteries to your liver. • Autoimmune conditions, inflam- mation, chronic liver disease • Associated with angina pectoris and myocardial infarction, diabetes mellitus, lack of exercise, obesity, smoking, hypertension, and incomplete diet.

Test	Functional Range	Result	High/Low	Weakness/ Possibilities
LDL CHOLESTEROL	Less than 120 mg/dl		Normal High	The "bad" cholesterol, responsible for plaque build-up in the arteries. • Blood sugar problems, sugar & saturated fat eaters, stress related, increase risk of heart and small vessel diseases, poor exercise habits
CHOL/HDL RATIO	Less than 3.1		Normal High	It is the ratio between these substances that identify your risk of having heart problems. The lower the ratio, the safer you are. • Increased risk of having heart problems. **However, the Triglyceride/HDL ratio is best**.
TSH	1.8 – 3.0 uIU/ml		Normal High Low	TSH stimulates the thyroid gland to secrete additional T4 • Hypothyroid symptoms • Hyperthyroid symptoms (if less than 0.5)
FT3	3.0 – 4.0 pg/ml		Normal High Low	This test measures the free or active T3 hormone (unbound) levels, which is the actual hormones that culminates In an increase in metabolism and energy • Hyperthyroid symptoms • Hypothyroid symptoms

Test	Functional Range	Result	High/Low	Weakness/ Possibilities
FT4	– 1.5 ng/dl		Normal High Low	The measure of active T4 in the blood but, must be converted to T3 to impact metabolism • Hyperthyroid symptoms • Hypothyroid symptoms
T4, TOTAL	6—12 mcg/dl		Normal High Low	Reflects the total output of the thyroid gland and actual T4 hormone released • Hyperthyroid symptoms • Hypothyroid symptoms
T3, TOTAL	60-180 ng/dl 0.6-1.81 ng/ml		Normal High Low	T3 is the most active thyroid hormone which is largely protein–bound but not necessarily available for metabolic activity • Hyperthyroid symptoms • Hypothyroid symptoms
REVERSE T3	25-30 ng/dl		Normal High Low	Your body, especially the liver, can constantly be converting T4 to RT3 as a way to get rid of any unneeded T4 • Hypothyroidism symptoms • Hypothyroid symptoms
T3 UPTAKE	28 -38 mg/dL		Normal High Low	Indirect measurement of unsaturated binding sites on the thyroid binding proteins • Hyperthyroid symptoms • Hypothyroid symptoms

Test	Functional Range	Result	High/Low	Weakness/ Possibilities
TPO AB	Above lab range 0-34		Normal	Check in cases of autoimmune thyroid disorders
TGB AB	Above lab range 0-40		Normal	Check in cases of autoimmune thyroid disorders
TH. BIND GLOB	18-27		Normal	This test measures the amount of proteins in the blood that transport thyroid hormones to the cells. Inherited thyroxine-binding globulin deficiency is a genetic condition that typically does not cause any health problems.
FTI (Free Thyroxine Index)	1.2-4.9 mg/dL		Normal High Low	The amount of unbound, physiologically active thyroxine (T4) in serum • Hyperthyroidism • Hypothyroid, low levels of selenium
WBC	5.0 – 8.0		Normal High Low	Fight infection, immune system, found in bone marrow. Protects body against infection and inflammation • Acute stressed/ compromised immune system, infection • Chronic stressed/ compromised immune system, infection

Test	Functional Range	Result	High/Low	Weakness/ Possibilities
RBC	Female: 3.9 – 4.4 Male: 4.2 – 4.9		Normal High Low	Erythrocytes; relates to anemia. Red blood cells carry oxygen to the cells & carbon dioxide back to the lungs • Dehydration, Polycythemia (a blood disorder in which your bone marrow makes too many red blood cells), altitude sickness, emphysema • Anemias, iron deficiency, B12 needs, menses, Internal or external bleeding
HEMOGLOBIN	Female: 13.5 – 14.5 Male: 14 - 15		Normal High Low	The oxygen carrying molecule in red blood cells • Dehydration, Polycythemia (a blood disorder in which your bone marrow makes too many red blood cells), altitude sickness, emphysema • Menses or iron deficiency anemia, B6, B12, bleeding or loss of blood

Test	Functional Range	Result	High/Low	Weakness/ Possibilities
HEMATOCRIT	Female: 37 – 44 Male: 40 - 48		Normal High Low	Percentage of red blood cells to whole blood (plasma). Relates to abnormal state of hydration, also the spleen denoting the amount of blood cell breakdown. • Dehydration, Polycythemia (a blood disorder in which your bone marrow makes too many red blood cells), altitude sickness, emphysema • Low Vitamin B12/ Folic Acid, C, B1,B6, anemia, protein deficiency, improper diet, ulcerations, menses or iron deficiency anemias, bleeding or loss of blood
MCV	85 – 92 cu icrons		Normal High Low	Average volume of many cells. • Anemia - B12/ Folic acid deficiency • Iron deficiency, low B6, loss of blood
MCH	27 – 32 cu icrons		Normal High Low	A hemoglobin-RBC ratio, gives the weight of hemoglobin in an average red cell. Relates to iron anemia • Anemia - B12/ Folic acid deficiency • Anemia - Low B6, iron deficiency; need Vitamin C, internal bleeding

Test	Functional Range	Result	High/Low	Weakness/ Possibilities
MCHC	32 – 35%		Normal High Low	The volume of hemoglobin in an average red cell. Helps distinguish normal colored red cells from: • Anemia - B12/ Folic acid deficiency • Anemia - Low B6, iron deficiency, Need Vitamin C, internal bleeding
RD	Less than 13		Normal High	Indicator of red blood cell size. • B12/Folate anemia and iron anemia
PLATELETS	50,000 – 450,000		Normal High Low	Cells in blood that form clots. • Polycethemia, free radical pathways, infection disorders • Leukemia, immune dysfunction

Test	Functional Range	Result	High/Low	Weakness/ Possibilities
NEUTROPHILS	40 – 60%		Normal High Low	This is a type of white blood cell. Amount of infection fighting capacity. The "good guys" • Immune compromise, infections and poisonings, possible bacterial infection, excessive amount of foreign protein due to undigested protein and muscle breakdown. • Low immune, free radical pathways, deficient Vitamins A, B-6, B-12, folic acid, iron, and copper; toxin
LYMPHOCYTES	25 – 40%		Normal High Low	This is a type of white blood cell. Aids in the destruction and handling of body toxins & by-products of protein metabolism. Relates to the healing process • Stressed immune system, possible viral infection, hepatitis, fever, infection. • Low immune, free radical pathways

Test	Functional Range	Result	High/Low	Weakness/ Possibilities
MONOCYTES	Less than 7%		Normal High	This is a type of white blood cell. Formed in the spleen and bone marrow, they can ingest and digest large bacteria. Relates to normal tissue breakdown by the liver • Inflammation, infection, parasites, BPH, possible viral infection, possible arthritis, stress and insufficient liquids.
EOSINOPHILS If Monocytes are above 7 and Eosinophils are above 3, check for parasites	Less than 3%		Normal High	This is a type of white blood cell. Responsible for the protection and preservation of life via the immunologic response. Relates to infections, inflamma-tions, diseases and allergies • Parasites, allergy, food allergies, intestinal infection, skin disease.
BASOPHILS	0 – 1%		Normal High	This is a type of white blood cell. Involved in deep membrane allergies. Relates to the immune response, inflammation, and Gastrointestinal tract • Parasites, inflam-mation, possible allergies, hyper-thyroidism, stress, blood compli-cations E and C, blood clotting.

Test	Functional Range	Result	High/Low	Weakness/ Possibilities
CRP (cardio) C-reactive protein	<2.0			Patients with levels of CRP are at an increased risk of diabetes, hypertension and cardiovascular disease. This is a marker for inflammation. Patients with active autoimmune disease can have high numbers. **Be sure to get this below 2.** Use supplements that decrease inflammation • Lower relative cardiovascular risk
	2.0—3.0			• Average relative cardiovascular risk
	3.1—10.0			• Higher relative cardiovascular risk • *High Inflammation
Erythrocyte sedimentation rate.	Males: 0-15 Females: 0-20		High	Marker of non-specific tissue inflammation or destruction • Indication of a disease process going on.
VAP cholesterol analysis	Goal is to have large particle size			This is the best way to determine the particle distribution of cholesterol. If you are worried about your cholesterol levels, this is the test to have
Insulin Fasting	Goal is less than 10 IU/ml			Provides a view as to how the body manages blood sugar. High levels of insulin are inflammatory contributing to heart disease.

Test	Functional Range	Result	High/Low	Weakness/ Possibilities
Vitamin D3 25-Hydroxy	50-100 ng/ml SUFFICIENT; **Must be in this range if you have an autoimmune disease** 10-30 Insufficiency <10 ng/ml Deficient		Normal Low	Use to diagnose Vitamin D deficiency and monitor response to Vitamin D therapy. Controls the level of phosphate and calcium in blood; regulates bone health; **modulates the immune system**; regulates neuromuscular functions; plays a vital role in cardiovascular functions; balances blood sugar level and insulin production; promotes normal cellular growth • Fatigue, general muscle pain and weakness, muscle cramps, joint pain, chronic pain, mood swings and depression, weight gain, high blood pressure, restless sleep, poor concentration, headaches, bladder problems, constipation or diarrhea and weak immune system; rickets in children

Test	Functional Range	Result	High/Low	Weakness/ Possibilities
Homocysteine	<7 <7 is the goal		Normal	Homocysteine is an amino acid in the blood. Is another marker to monitor inflammation along with CRP. I use B vitamins to help correct. • Too much of it is related to a higher risk of coronary heart disease, stroke or vascular disease (fatty deposits in peripheral arteries) Higher levels of homocys-teine can cause thyroid resistance; inability for T3 to get into the cell
Fibrinogen	Below 350		High	Increased risk of atherosclerotic disease (plaque buildup in arteries); heart attack

** This chart is a guide for nutritional support information and to reinforce systemic and metabolic heath and is not intended as a diagnosis or treatment for any symptoms, conditions or disease.

always order and review any bloodwork performed on a patient and determine patterns from the functional ranges previously listed. Most of the tests that I order are the ones listed above and are a good baseline of tests. However, if the patient's history is unique, I might include a few more. If you don't have insurance, Direct Labs is a place to get lab testing. You can find them on the web. Obviously, it helps to have a doctor that you can work with to help guide you. If you plan on running tests on yourself and you discover abnormal lab values and you don't know what it means, be sure to consult with a doctor.

When I evaluate a thyroid patient, we want to assess how the thyroid is functioning. The goal would be to get the numbers within the functional range. It is important to first rule out Hashimoto's. If you are positive for Hashimoto's, we may require advanced testing to search for the antigen (triggers). The most common triggers for autoimmune disease are food proteins, infections, environmental toxins and heavy metals. Furthermore, research has shown that leaky gut can contribute to autoimmune disease. "Together with the gut-associated lymphoid tissue and the neuroendocrine network, the intestinal epithelial barrier, with its intercellular tight junctions, controls the equilibrium between tolerance and immunity to nonself-antigens." "When the finely tuned trafficking of macro-molecules is dysregulated in individuals, both intestinal and extraintestinal autoimmune disorders can occur." Nat. Clin. Pract. Gastroenterol. Hepatol. 2005 Sep: 2(9): 416-422. Mechanisms of Disease: The Role of Intestinal Barrier Function in the Pathogenesis of Gastrointestinal Autoimmune Diseases.

I use Cyrex Labs to test for food sensitivities and leaky gut. You can find them online at cyrexlabs.com. They offer different arrays of testing. I use the Gluten Array 3, Leaky gut Array 2 and the Cross Reactive Array 4. I also use ELISA/ACT Biotechnologies as they offer testing that covers an extensive variety of foods including chemicals, preservatives, medications, additives, molds and metals.

If you have an autoimmune disease, we need to look for the triggers and repair leaky gut. These advanced tests become beneficial.

I use stool testing to check for gut infections, parasites, yeast, dysbiosis and normal function. Genova Diagnostics offers some useful tests.

To assess adrenal function and hormones, I use Diagnostechs and BioHealth. I prefer using salivary tests to monitor adrenal function and hormones. If you use blood testing for hormones, be sure get free hormones checked also.

Spectracell offers micronutrient/nutritional testing.

Vitamin, mineral and antioxidant deficiencies have been shown to suppress the functions of the immune system. You may be deficient in some vitamins, minerals, antioxidants and/or other essential micronutrients and not even know about it. The thyroid needs nutrients to function properly and this is one way to find out what you need.

Doctors Data "24-hour iodine/iodide load test" has become a useful analysis for practitioners to determine iodine needs. Doctors Data can also be used for the assessment of retention of toxic metals in the body and the status of essential nutrient elements. Toxic metals do not have any useful physiological function and can adversely affect virtually every organ.

I do not order all tests on all patients. It depends on the information I feel I need to help me change what I will do for them. Again, this is where having someone working with you will save you a lot of trial and error.

Where can you start? Obviously, start with the information and guidelines I outlined in the Diet chapter. In addition, I will outline some protocols that you can use. These protocols are designed to give the body the nutrients it needs to repair from specific issues. Diet alone may not be enough.

The foundation of any holistic approach to health begins with repairing gut function. You can

always benefit from gut repair.

Repairing Gut Function

Hashimoto's Disease - With any autoimmune disease, leaky gut must be corrected (see below). In addition, your Vitamin D level needs to be between 60-80. Take between 5,000-10,000 per day and retest in 8-12 weeks. Fish oil EPA and DHA, probiotics and glutathione are used to modulate the immune system. If you can determine whether your TH1 or TH2 is dominant, use supplements to help. Detox your body of any toxins and take steps to manage any possible viral or bacterial infections.

Graves Disease - Graves is also an autoimmune disease. Follow the guidelines I listed for Hashimoto's. In addition, 2-5 grams of L-carnitine can calm the hyperactive thyroid in addition to a product called Thyrocalm for hyperthyroid.

Addressing leaky gut - You need to follow the autoimmune diet described in the Diet section. If you have an autoimmune disease, you should start with this. The time for repair will vary with patients as it can take anywhere from 1-6 months. If you tested for leaky gut, you would have a way of tracking your progress. If not and you have autoimmune disease, do it for 12 weeks as mentioned. The supplements I use are GI Revive from Designs For Health or Repairvite from Apex.

If you have gut infections, parasites or yeast, I will use Micob X from Designs For Health or GI Synergy from Apex. I also will use a probiotic with a dose of 50-100 billion. This would be done for a period of 12 weeks, monitored with a stool test.

Hypochlorhydria – This should be suspected if your total protein, globulin and albumin are out of the functional ranges (high or low), if you have burping and bloating problems, gas after meals or difficulty digesting fruits. You may have low stomach acid and would then need to take HCL to help restore good stomach acid. I recommend HCL Prozyme from Apex or HCL from Premier Research Labs. If you use antacids and have pain after eating along with heartburn, excessive acid production is a problem which is a result of low stomach acid to begin with. Without sufficient amounts of stomach acid, when food enters the stomach, it will remain in the stomach and begins to ferment. This creates the excessive acid that causes pain. Taking HCL at this point would make things worse. Start with MSM from Designs For Health and or Gastro ULC from Apex. After correcting the problem, you would proceed to increase acid levels to normal with HCL.

Adrenal Glands - If you have difficulty staying asleep or falling asleep, crave salt, suffer from fatigue in the mornings and afternoons, have mid-afternoon headaches, excessive perspiration and/or weight gain, your adrenal glands might be stressed or fatigued. For adrenal support, use Adaptocrine from Apex. Phosphorylated serine is also used to balance the Cortisol levels. However, the biggest stressor to the adrenal glands is unstable blood sugar. To fix the adrenals, you have to manage blood sugar.

Reactive hypoglycemic (low blood sugar) – Craving sweets, having blurred vision, being irritable between meals, needing coffee to function or being lightheaded, shaky, jittery, nervous or easily agitated. If these symptoms are a problem, you will need to manage them with small, frequent meals. Be sure to have a protein-based breakfast. You can use essential fatty acids and Proglyco-SP from Apex. This may need to be done in conjunction with supporting the adrenal glands. If your fasting blood sugar is below 85 and your LDH is below 140 and you have the above symptoms, you are most likely a reactive hypoglycemic.

High Blood Sugar - Fatigue after meals, craving sweets, cravings for sugar, must have dessert, frequent urination, increased thirst and weight gain. In addition, if your fasting blood sugar is above 100 and your hemoglobin A1C is above 5.7, your cells are becoming resistant to insulin and blood sugar is on the rise. Excess blood sugar and insulin are inflammatory and will lead to cardiovascular complications. I use the Maintenance Diet I described in the Diet section along with Omega 3 fatty acids, EPA and DHA (fish oil). I will also use a product called Glysen after meals from Apex.

If it has been determined that you have dysglycemia or reactive hypoglycemia, I suggest that you eat something every 2-3 hours. This helps to maintain stable blood sugar throughout the day and prevents Cortisol (from your adrenal glands) and other stress hormones like epinephrine and norepinephrine from being released whenever your blood sugar begins to drop. Follow these rules:

1. Breakfast is to consist solely of animal protein. Sardines make the best first meal due to their high Omega 3

content and high protein yield. There is a lot of energy in a can of sardines (the ones that are in olive oil are the best and only ones I know of that are safe for us to eat). You can eat as much as you want and any type animal protein, as long as it does not contain any of the forbidden foods or spices.

2. 1-2 hours after your first meal, you may eat your carbo-hydrate and protein meal. I usually eat what I had for dinner the night before, or you may eat another breakfast with buckwheat or mixed vegetables.

3. 2-3 hours later could be your lunch, which is any of the approved vegetables along with animal based protein.

4. 2-3 hours later: meat and vegetables again (any and as much as you like).

5. 2-3 hours later: meat and vegetables (all you can eat).

6. An hour or so before you go to bed, eat a small meal consisting of mostly protein (at least 85%) and the rest vegetables.

Here are a few tips that will also help:

- Snack on stone fruits (fruits with pits) and fresh vegetables throughout the day, if needed.

- If you can't eat it, you shouldn't put it in your hair or on your skin. So, if soap contains soy or wheat or milk products, then you cannot use that soap (or lotion, make-up, etc.)

- Stay away from deep fried foods. Bake or stir-fry your meals instead

- Choose lots of colorful vegetables and especially lots of green, leafy ones

- Breakfast is to consist solely of animal protein. It can be as much as you want and any type, as long as it does not contain any of the forbidden foods or spices.

- Your meals are to always have at least some protein

from animal sources if possible. Saturated fats are your friend; we are made of saturated fats. Try and remember that your brain, nerves, myelin and sex hormones are made of cholesterol. Each cell in your body produces its own cholesterol so don't let junk science into your head or believe that you are going to have high cholesterol because you eat meat.

- Drink plenty of water throughout the day. You may add fresh squeezed lemon to the water for added flavor; however, no juices or sugar is to be added.

- Remember that you have to eat to live now, not live to eat. It may be rough at first but take it one day at a time. Do not let this overwhelm you and make you quit. I assure you that once you get over the 'hump', you will see that this is all worthwhile!

Go to http://www.ceceliasmarketplace.com/gluten-free-casein-free-soy-free-guide/ and purchase the *Gluten/Casein/Soy Free Grocery Shopping Guide*. Always read labels, even if you buy it often because you never know if the ingredients have been changed.

The easiest way to follow the initial portion of your program is to only eat MEAT & VEGETABLES!

References:

i. http://www.nongmoproject.org/learn-more/what-is-gmo/

ii. 2 EPA-823-R-04-0053; *Binding of Insulin Receptors to Lectins: Evidence for Common Carbohydrate Determinants on Several Membrane Receptors*: Jose A. Hedo, Len C. Harrison, Jesse Roth, Biochemistry, 1981, 20 (12), pp 3385–3393; DOI: 10.1021/bi00515a013: Publication Date: June 1981

Detoxification - Vitamin C Flush

The Vitamin C flush can be useful to detoxify toxins (bacteria, environmental, heavy metals, medications) from the body. It has been researched with good results. It will also boost your immune system as it saturates the cells with vitamin C. Everyone has had some exposure to toxins so this can be useful. If you are TH1 dominant, do not perform this test. If you feel worse, you need to stop taking Vitamin C. Chances are you are TH2 dominant.

Directions:

a) Start on an empty stomach and dissolve ½-1 tsp. of Vitamin C buffered powder mixed with 4-8 oz. water or juice. Allow the effervescence to subside, then drink.

b) Keep a log of the time and amount consumed.

c) Repeat every 15 minutes until you have watery diarrhea (don't stop with gas or loose stools, they should be watery), then stop taking the Vitamin C. If after 4 doses you do not feel a rumble in the tummy, double the dose.

d) Keep track of the amount it took to saturate your tissues. Your regular, daily dose will be 50-75% of this amount and it should be taken daily, in a divided dose.

Your daily dose is a place to start, however your needs will change. For best results do the flush weekly for 1 month, then monthly. This is a great way to boost the immune system for cold and flu season.

Which Ascorbate (Vitamin C) Is Best to Use?

It is preferable to use a 100% l-ascorbate, fully reduced, buffered mineral ascorbate form of Vitamin C that contains a proper balance of the major essential buffering minerals: potassium, magnesium, calcium, and zinc.

When doing the flush, be sure to use 2,000-3,000 grams per serving which will be a ½ or 1 full teaspoon. I use buffered Vitamin C from Designs For Health and Perque Buffered Ascorbate Powder. Perque has a very detailed protocol and explanation if needed.

If you have Anemia

If you are anemic, you want to rule out that you don't have uterine fibroids, cysts or anything that could be causing low blood volume. Red blood cells, hemoglobin, hematocrit, MCV, MCHC, iron and ferritin will all be low. If that is not the case, your anemia would be of a different form. This could require the help of a professional to determine the type. I do consult with many patients that are on iron supplements. When asked why they are supplementing, they mention that their iron is low. Before taking any iron supplements, you need to have low serum iron and saturation, high TIBS and low ferritin. Ferritin is the storage form of iron and is very important in determining iron deficiency. If ferritin is low, you can consider iron supplementation. I also use B vitamins with some anemia cases.

The Liver

The liver has many important functions. To name a few, it:

- Detoxifies toxic chemicals, infections, intestinal microbes and alcohol
- It produces proteins involved with protein metabolism
- Regulates blood sugar levels
- Controls the production of hormone (converts T4 to T3).

Some symptoms of liver dysfunction are: coated tongue, bad breath, red palms and hands, reddish face from increased facial blood vessels, acne, rosacea, nausea, dark circles under eyes, rashes, itchy skin and brownish spots and blemishes on skin.

Foods that protect and detoxify the liver include: apples, beets, carrots, onions, garlic, eggs, brown rice, broccoli, spinach, cauliflower, cabbage, brussel sprouts and grape-fruit. It would also be helpful to juice vegetables daily. I also suggest a fiber supplement that binds to toxins and helps eliminate them. I use Galactan from Premier Research Labs.

Supplements - B vitamins are a must. I use Max B, a live source from Premier Research Labs, Vitamin C, Vitamin E, selenium and zinc.

Herbs: Milk thistle, artichoke leaf, turmeric.

The coffee enema has also been used to detoxify the liver. Caffeine allows the liver to empty its contents into the colon. Premier Research Labs sells a kit with instructions and the coffee to be used for the enema. Be sure to repair gut function before the coffee enema. If you decide to do this quality product, it is important to use Premier Research Labs. I have patients that have felt wonderful after this protocol. It would not be a bad Idea to do this once a year for maintenance.

I have also used rectal suppositories that have organic coffee along with a few other useful detoxifiers.

Is Your Body pH balanced?

You get your cholesterol tested. You get your blood pressure tested. Just like your cholesterol and blood pressure, your pH says a lot about the state of your health. It tells you how acidic or alkaline your tissues and fluids are. Your pH affects all aspects of your well-being. In order to test your pH, you will need to purchase some pH strips and check your first morning urine (midstream). Record the results. Your first morning urine should be between 6.4 and 7.0. The goal is to have consistent readings between 6.4 and 7.0 for two weeks.

Symptoms of being acidic include:

- Poor digestion
- Low energy
- Inability to lose weight
- Increased aches and pain - "inflammation"
- Decreased minerals
- Body will leach minerals out of bone to buffer blood, leading to osteoporosis
- Greater risk for heavy metal toxicity and increased free radicals
- Increase colds and flu due to welcoming environment for viruses and bacteria
- It irritates all organs it comes in contact with, especially thyroid

The Pink Salt Flush: Intestinal Cleansing

Think of a salt flush as a very thorough colonic. Where a colonic only cleanses the colon, a salt flush cleanses the colon as well as the stomach and small intestines. A salt flush is prepared by mixing 1 teaspoon of Premier Pink Salt into 16 ounces of warm purified water. It is the easiest intestinal cleanse ever. The best time to do a salt flush is first thing in the morning when you have easy access to a bathroom.

The exit of the stomach into the small intestines is on the lower right hand side of the stomach. When you drink it, the saltwater goes to the bottom of the stomach, below the opening. After drinking the saltwater on an empty stomach, lie on your right side for 30 minutes to "tip the teapot," insuring that the saltwater goes out of the stomach and directly into the intestinal tract. The opening from the stomach into the small intestines looks like a teapot spout. Once the saltwater is in the small intestines, the muscle contractions will carry it down the rest of the way. In about an hour, you should be able to massage the left hand side of your lower abdomen and hear liquids gurgling. These are liquids that have flowed into the large intestine almost ready for evacuation.

A Salt Flush gives most people a rapid, full bowel elimination within 30 to 60 minutes and may possibly stimulate a secondary bowel elimination two or more hours later. If no flush occurs, it may indicate that a person is salt-deficient. In this case, simply continue the salt flush once per day anyway. Continue salt flushing daily for about two weeks, then once per week, while you are undergoing a detoxification program. Your practitioner may ask you to increase the amount of salt you are using during the flushes.

Water retention rarely occurs with salt flushes. If this occurs, simply discontinue the salt flushes for a few days then begin again. You may need additional kidney nutritional support.

The objective of the salt flush is to send water down the intestinal tract. Sometimes the saltwater does not flow into the intestinal tract properly. For best results, drink the recommended saltwater solution and then lie on your right side for 30 minutes. This ensures that the saltwater will quickly leave the stomach and go into the small intestines.

One of the best ways to cleanse the body rapidly and efficiently is to do a salt flush and then follow it with a Premier Coffee Enema. For most people, the salt flush will elicit a second mild purging of the GI tract within 2 hours. After the flush occurs (a healthy bowel elimination), prepare a Premier Coffee Enema (PCE). The preparation time for a PCE is about 15 to 20 minutes. The goal of every PCE is to retain it for about 10 minutes. Since all the blood passes through the liver every 3 minutes, you will be able to cleanse your entire blood supply three times a session.

The major benefit of doing a PCE after a Pink Salt Flush is that the flush first clears the colon of fecal debris lower in the tract. Then all the beneficial alkaloids and compounds from the fresh ground, quantum-state coffee can be most efficiently absorbed via the intestinal wall into the blood for maximum cleansing of the liver and gallbladder system.

This combo can be used daily or weekly until desired results are achieved. A monthly or quarterly maintenance schedule can be implemented for peak performance for the digestive system and whole body health.

Salt Flush Guidelines

A person weighing from 90 to 170 lbs. - use 1 tsp. Premier Pink Salt (see below) in

16 oz. water

A person weighing 171 to 200 lbs. - use 1 ½ tsp. Premier Pink Salt in 16 oz. water

A person weighing 201 to 230 lbs. or more - use 2 tsp. Premier Pink Salt in 16 oz. water

Thyroid Support

You can't have a discussion of thyroid support without discussing iodine. Should you or shouldn't you use Iodine? I will say that if you have thyroid nodules, iodine can make matters worse. If you have Hashimoto's, proceed with caution. I have consulted with patients who had their thyroid problems get worse after self-medicating with iodine. I have also consulted with patients that have used iodine and it has helped immensely. My approach is to fix the underlying physiological problems first--gut dysfunction, blood sugar and adrenals, immune function, liver, detox, anemia and infections. If the patient has not significantly improved at this point, I would consider iodine support. With most this does not happen. When I do I use Iodine, I use a product from Premier Research Labs called Xenostat or Thyroven with which I have had no problems.

Doctors Data has an iodine loading test that allows you to determine if your body is deficient in iodine. If you have researched thyroid long enough, you will notice that there are two sides to this iodine position. Both sides make valid claims and sound arguments. My job as a doctor is to get patients better and consider what is necessary for the individual patient. I have to set aside any position or stance of being pro or against iodine. I can only speak from experience as I have stated above and I hope it helps.

Body Temperature and Thyroid

Normal body temperature is 98.6 and should occur mid-day. Morning temperature should be between 97.8 and 98.2. Patients with hypothyroidism will have consistently low body temperatures. Patients who have body temperatures that fluctuate from low to high would indicate that the adrenal glands are involved.

In addition to lab testing, monitoring body temperatures give us a measuring stick to see if we are improving the adrenals and thyroid function. It could also be a useful pretest to see if adrenals and hormones are involved in the problem.

To test your body temperature, take your temperature as soon as you get out of bed and record the number. Alternatively, take your temperature every 3 hours starting with the morning and record the daily average. As you start to accumulate more readings, you may see some patterns develop.

Gallbladder Flush

<u>Days</u>

1-5   Drink 1 quart of organic apple juice. Eat normally

6   Drink as much of your quart of organic apple juice before noon as you can. Eat a normal lunch. At 3:00 and 5:00 p.m., drink an Epsom salt laxative (the directions are on the box. The only change is to use fresh squeezed orange juice instead of water). Eat only citrus for dinner. At bedtime, mix ½ cup of cold-pressed olive oil with ½ cup of lemon juice and drink. Lie down on your right side with your right knee pulled up to your chest for 30 minutes.

Beginning at some point the next day, you should see stones in your stool. Stones look greenish in color and can vary in size from the size of a grape seed to the size of a grape. The smaller stones seem to be darker in color. It can take a few days to clear them all out if you have very many. Take a natural laxative during this time to help prevent having an attack. Even mild constipation can contribute to a gallbladder attack. This flush should be repeated in 30 days if you see any stones.

Notes: Cold-pressed Olive oil varies greatly in taste. The ones that are greenish have a very strong flavor. You can warm the oil just a tiny bit so it's not as thick

Kidney Stone flush

Coke/Asparagus Remedy:

This is the only time that I'd ever recommend that someone drink a Coke. Why? This procedure works pretty consistently. If the stones are less than 5 mm., it will turn them into fine sand and pass painlessly. Items needed:

- 2-Liter bottle of Coke Classic - **NOTE**: It MUST be Coke Classic. Pepsi and all other types of soda won't work.
- Bowl of fresh asparagus

PROCEDURE:

- Drink the entire 2-liter bottle of Coke in less than two hours. Horrible for blood sugar, but it's only once.
- About 20 minutes before you are done with the Coke, boil the bowl of asparagus. As soon as you are done with the Coke, eat the entire bowl of asparagus. If it does the job, you will pass the stone painlessly within a few hours.

Water is Key

Water is the pillar of life. Our life and our health are completely dependent upon water. It manages all functions of our body, from metabolism to cognition. It is not only important for our physical body but is also responsible for our thought processes. (Our brains are 90% water.)

Beyond its biophysical life-giving effect, water is also chemically a solvent, transporter and cleanser. Throughout metabolism, it facilitates cleansing, the transport of nutrients and the removal of waste products. It maintains the osmotic pressure of the cells and regulates the body temperature. All metabolic procedures rely on water to function. The same is true for extracting toxins though the kidneys, the colon, the skin and the lungs.

On a daily basis the human body discharges about 0.4 to 0.6 gallons of water. This perpetual loss of liquid needs to be constantly replenished! The amount of water our body needs depends on our weight. Drink about ½ an ounce of water per pound of body weight per day. For example: if you weigh 130 lbs., you need to be drinking 65 ounces of water per day. That is pure water ... not coffee, tea, wine, beer or soda which dehydrate your body. The fewer ingredients (including minerals) the water contains the better because water has a flushing function. Mineral water or "carbonated water" is saturated and can no longer absorb toxins.

And do not drink tap water. Tap water is full of fluoride and chlorine which compete with the iodine molecule in the thyroid. Your thyroid runs your metabolism. It is the "gas pedal" of the body so iodine is needed to make thyroid hormones!

Pure spring water is best.

Adequate daily intake of high quality water is of paramount importance. With the starvation of the body for water comes the expiration of our cells. The more our bodies are starved for water, the greater the number of cells that will die. Dehydration follows, and the process of

aging is accelerated.

DETOX With Infrared Sauna Therapy

Sweating is the body's safe and natural way to heal and detox. Sweat carries toxins out of the body and pushes it through the pores. Waste is also removed via urine and feces. Sweating helps the body release heat and keeps your internal core temperature as consistent as needed. The average person has 2.6 million sweat glands. Sweat glands are distributed over the majority of the human body. Skin is the largest organ in the body and it plays a significant part in the detox process.

Detoxing using a Sunlight Sauna is 7 to 10 times greater than a conventional sauna. In a Sunlight Sauna, the average person sweats out 20% toxins and 80% water! In a conventional sauna, the average person sweats out 3% toxins and 97% water.

Far-Infrared Saunas are what I recommend. You may have some studios in your area where you can buy sessions. Saunas are also available to purchase for your home. Use the Infrared that mimics the sun.

Why Detoxify?

Detox can be helpful for people suffering from thyroid conditions. If you have Hashimoto's, your immune system may be reacting to a biotoxin or a metal. By detoxifying the body you are going to rid these potential triggers, stopping the attack on the thyroid.

Detoxifying can help:

- Allergies
- Depression
- Low blood sugar
- Anxiety
- Headaches
- Digestive disorders
- Arthritis
- Heart disease
- Mental illness
- Asthma
- High cholesterol
- Obesity
- Chronic infections

Detox therapy is also useful for those suffering from immune system problems that include chronic fatigue syndrome, environmental illness/multiple chemical sensitivity and fibromyalgia. It is interesting to note that more than 90%

of the patients that I see with fibromyalgia have an under-lying thyroid problem.

Therefore, detox has also become a prominent treatment as people have become more aware of it. It is estimated that one in every four Americans suffers from some level of heavy metal poisoning, including mercury, lead, cadmium and aluminum.

Toxins in the body also include chemical pollutants such as pesticides, DDT, PCB (polychlorinatedbiphenyls) and food additives. Drugs and alcohol also have toxic effects in the body.

Source: Sweat It All Out; How Stuff Works; Zane R. Gard, MD & Erma J. Brown, BSN, PhN TlfDP, October 1992

Organic Food

In the U.S., everyone has choices to make in terms of what type of food they will eat and how it will affect their health. The question becomes: Do you want to sacrifice your current and future health for convenience and taste or choose more expensive, healthy foods and cut back in other areas?

The Most Important Foods to Buy - Organic

If you're on a tight budget but want to improve your diet by shopping organic, animal products like meat, poultry and eggs is the place to start. Since animal products tend to bio-accumulate toxins from their pesticide-laced feed, concentrating them in far higher concentrations than are typically present in vegetables, it is strongly recommended you buy organically raised meats.

Unlike conventional fruits and vegetables, where peeling

and washing can sometimes reduce the amount of these toxins, the pesticides and drugs that these animals get exposed to during their lives can become incorporated into their very tissues, especially their fat. While you can cut off some of it, you may still be ingesting high amounts of toxins if you consume such foods regularly. Another important factor that sets organic meat apart from its conventional counterpart is it will not contain antibiotics and other growth-promoting drugs.

When choosing organic beef, take the additional step to make certain the cows are exclusively grass-fed. This can make a big difference in the quality, taste, and nutrient content of the beef.

For chickens, it would be important to make sure they are cage-free, or free-range, chickens, as well as being organic. And eggs from truly organic, pastured chickens are FAR less likely to contain dangerous bacteria such as salmonella, and their nutrient content is also much higher than commercially raised eggs.

Dairy: Is Organic Worth It?

Organic dairy products are important because they'll be free from pesticides and Monsanto's genetically engineered growth hormone rBGH. However, the real issue is not organic vs. non- organic milk, but pasteurized vs. non-pasteurized, or raw, milk.

Hands down, raw milk, even not organic, is the superior choice.

Pasteurization transforms the physical structure of the proteins in milk, such as casein, and alters the shape of the amino acid configuration into a foreign protein that your body is not

equipped to handle. The process also destroys the friendly bacteria found naturally in milk and drastically reduces the micronutrient and vitamin content.

Pasteurization destroys part of the Vitamin C in raw

milk, encourages the growth of harmful bacteria and turns milk's naturally occurring sugar (lactose) into beta-lactose. Beta-lactose is rapidly absorbed in the human body with the result that hunger can return quickly after a glass of milk--especially in children.

The pasteurization process also makes most of the calcium found in raw milk insoluble. This can lead to a host of health problems in children, among them rickets and bad teeth. And then there's the destruction of about 20 percent of the iodine available in raw milk which can cause constipation. Raw milk contains good bacteria that are essential for a healthy digestive system, and offers protection against disease-causing bacteria.

When pasteurized milk is also homogenized, a substance known as xanthine oxidase is created. This compound can play a role in oxidative stress by acting as a free radical in your body.

Which Organic Produce Should You Buy?

In terms of pesticides, the Environmental Working Group has done the work for you and identified the 12 fruits and vegetables with the highest pesticide load, making them the most important to buy or grow organic:

The Dirty Dozen List:

- Peaches
- Apples
- Sweet bell peppers
- Celery
- Nectarines
- Strawberries
- Cherries
- Lettuce
- Grapes (imported)

- Pears
- Spinach
- Potatoes

Meanwhile, the produce below has the lowest pesticide load when conventionally grown. Consequently, they are the safest conventionally grown crops to consume:

- Broccoli
- Eggplant
- Cabbage
- Banana
- Kiwi
- Asparagus
- Sweet peas (frozen)
- Mango
- Pineapple
- Sweet corn (frozen)
- Avocado
- Onion

Making Sure Your Organic Foods are Really Healthy

Ninety percent of the money Americans spend on food is spent on processed foods, which is a disaster for your health even if you're buying "organic" processed foods.

Just because someone slaps an organic label on a food product, that label does not somehow magically transform a junk food into a health food. Organic processed foods -- ice cream, potato chips, soda, etc. -- are just as detrimental to your health as conventional processed foods.

So when planning your food budget, make sure your organic choices are centered on whole foods like meat, raw dairy and produce -- not processed imposters.

Juicing 101

What Are the Benefits of Juicing?

First off, cooking and processing food destroys micronutrients by altering their shape and chemical composition. While eating cooked food that is nutritious is not entirely 'bad' for you, getting your veggies in primarily cooked form is not the desirable way to receive all of the amazing micronutrients from plants. This is especially true for those with advanced disease and impaired digestion. Plant fiber is excellent, and we still recommend that you incorporate it into your daily menu, yet adding fresh juice to the mix dramatically increases your nutrient intake. Raw vegetable juices furnish your body with live enzymes, bioactive vitamins, minerals and trace minerals that are otherwise decreased and destroyed by cooking.

Another thing to take into consideration is that it is pretty difficult to receive these micronutrient gems from raw veggies because of our inability to fully masticate (chew) raw plant fiber. Therefore, a lot of vitamins, proteins and minerals stay locked in the plant fiber as it moves through the intestinal tract.

What are some of these nutrients? Amino acids, which form the building blocks for protein; soluble fiber that helps control bad cholesterol; essential fatty acids that the body cannot make on its own, yet which are essential to healthy nerve cells and form part of the cellular membrane around all cells; phyto-chemicals that give plants their unique colors, tastes, and scents, and which have anti-oxidant and anti-carcinogenic properties; minerals, such as calcium, potassium, iron, and zinc, that are essential to proper cell functioning; enzymes, which aid in digestion and regulate chemical reactions in the body, and last but not least – vitamins, vitamins, vitamins! Fruit and vegetable juices contain Vitamins A, C, D, E, K, as well as B- complex vitamins, all essential to maintaining good health.

Why Juice? Top Reasons

There are many reasons why you will want to consider incorporating vegetable juicing into your optimal health program:

1. Juicing helps you absorb all the nutrients from the vegetables. This is important because most of us have impaired digestion as a result of making less-than-optimal food choices over many years. This limits our ability to break down and absorb nutrients. Juicing literally helps to "pre-digest" them for you, so you will receive most of the nutrition.

2. Juicing allows you to consume an optimal amount of vegetables in an efficient manner. How many of us can realistically and consistently incorporate a wide variety of plant foods (6-8 servings) into our daily lives? Not many. It can become time consuming and frustrating, but it can be easily accomplished with a quick glass of vegetable juice.

3. You can add a wider variety of vegetables to your diet. Many people eat the same vegetables or salads every day. Juicing provides you the opportunity to include a wide variety of vegetables that you may not normally enjoy eating whole.

4. Juicing helps reduce over acidity in the blood and improves your pH. Due to many years of poor dietary habits, most people tend to be on the acidic side. Meat, dairy, processed grains, sugars, sports drinks,

soft drinks, alcohol, etc. are all very acidic. Vegetable juices are highly alkaline and improve your blood pH. This is why so many feel energized after drinking vegetable juice. It is like a shot of oxygen which helps to maintain balanced pH for optimal health. Balanced pH is key to optimal health.

5. Juicing can help reverse disease. Alkalizing minerals from vegetable sources help to restore the alkaline and mineral balance in the cells. They speed the recovery from disease by supporting the body's own healing response and cell regeneration. The added oxygen and micronutrients also help to rebuild the blood.

6. Kids can fall in love with juices. There are a million ways to make vegetable juice, and usually with the addition of fresh fruit, a child's pallet can be rewired. Adding beets also masks the green look.

But Wait, Can't I Just Buy Juice From the Store?

Not unless that store has a juice bar. Fruit and vegetable juice that is pressed and stored in bottles begins the process of oxidation as soon as it comes in contact with oxygen, and a major loss of nutrients begins to occur. It is typically recommended that you drink a juice within 20 minutes of preparing it; this is when the nutrients are most intact. Therefore, even when juicing, it is not recommended to save juices in the fridge after making one. Just down it! Here are some ideas for combining fruits and vegetables:

a) Carrot and Green Apples Are a Great Combination

One of the most pleasant combinations to begin with is carrots and green apples. You can never go wrong with carrots. They are especially beneficial for colon health and are a rich source of vitamin A, which is essential to the health of all the mucous membranes of the body. It is great for cleansing and detoxifying, too. You can add spinach or kale to this drink as well, and try it with lemon, too.

b) Cucumbers and Celery as Your Base

Cucumbers and celery are perfect as a base for a green juice. Cucumbers are an excellent source of Vitamin C, and celery is high in minerals (especially potassium) and B vitamins. Both are highly alkalizing and cleansing. They are full of water, and have a kind flavor. A cucumber and celery cocktail with a little apple or pear is a nice way to ease yourself in. Organic cucumbers are okay to juice with the skin on, but conventional cucumbers should be peeled. Try this combination: 1 cucumber, 4 celery stalks, 2 apples, 6-8 kale leaves and ½ lemon.

c) Organic Veggies

Juicing is for alkalizing, detoxifying, and purifying. Juicing veggies and fruits coated in pesticides kind of defeats your purpose. Try your best to get as much organic produce for your juicing as possible. Many of the staples for juicing are actually laced with the most pesticides, such as apples, celery, and greens. See the Dirty Dozen for the top 12 fruits and veggies with the most pesticides.

d) Low Glycemic Fruit is a Better Choice

While you can certainly juice fruits, if you are overweight, have cancer, high blood pressure, diabetes or other degenerative disease it is best to limit using fruits. The added sugar, although natural, may pose metabolic complications. Stick to low glycemic foods like pears or apples. Lemon and limes are good too because they have virtually no sugar. Additionally, lemons or limes are amazing at eliminating the bitter taste of the dark deep leafy green vegetables that provide most of the benefits of juicing.

Small amounts of more sugary fruit are okay from time to time, as long as you use small amounts. The ideal ratio should be 3:1 - three veggies to one piece of fruit.

Take Your Juice on an Empty Stomach

The best time for juicing is on an empty stomach, especially first thing in the morning. Make sure to "chew" your juice to activate enzymes in your saliva. Avoid gulping it down. Wait at least 30-45 minutes after your juice before taking in solid food.

It's Important to Listen to Your Body

It is very important to listen to your body when juicing. Your stomach should feel good all morning long. Though many people first come to juicing seeking help for a specific ailment or condition, there is no need to wait for something to go wrong before you try it! The human body has a remarkable capacity to fight disease, to heal, and even to renew itself. When you give it the nutrients it needs, it will respond in amazing ways, rewarding you by regulating your weight, increasing your levels of energy, fighting the effects of time, and even reducing your need to conventionally medicate conditions such as high blood pressure, metabolism and even acne. The cleansing power of juice makes it clear that the body knows what it is doing. Adding the good stuff helps get rid of the bad.

Why You Should Go Grain-Free

1. Grains aren't good for your gut.

   Intestinal health is critical to your overall health. If your gut isn't healthy, you can't absorb nutrients from the foods you eat. If you can't absorb nutrients from the foods you eat, your body is malnourished and is more prone to disease. Grains are associated with a condition called leaky gut syndrome. Tiny particles of grains, when ingested, can slip through the intestinal walls causing an immune response. With your immune system excessively taxed by constantly attacking these out-of-place particles of grain, it cannot effectively fight against true threats like pathogens.

2. You're probably gluten-intolerant.

If you're white, there's a good chance that you're gluten-intolerant to some degree. Current research estimates that about 1% of the population suffers from celiac disease, an auto- immune condition related to the ingestion of gluten-containing grains like wheat and barley; however, some researchers of celiac disease and gluten intolerance estimate that 30-40% of people of European descent are gluten-intolerant to some degree. That's a lot of people who are regularly consuming a food that makes them sick.

3. Grains cause inflammation.

Due to high starch content, grains are inflammatory foods. The more refined the grain, the more inflammatory it is. For example, unbleached white flour is more inflammatory than whole grain flour; however, whole grains are still moderately inflammatory foods and certainly more inflammatory than other foods like fresh vegetables and wholesome fats. Chronic inflammation is linked to a myriad of degenerative, modern diseases including arthritis, allergies, asthma, cardiovascular disease, bone loss, emotional imbalance and even cancer.

4. Grains are fairly new on the scene.

Prior to the advent of agriculture, humans relied on hunting and gathering for their foods. They foraged for wild greens, berries, fruits and other plants. They hunted wild animals. They fished for wild fish. They didn't plant a garden, or grow any amber waves of grain or, for that matter, drink dairy from domesticated animals since there simply wasn't any domesticated animals. Humans survived like this from the development of the appearance of the first Homo sapiens about 47,000 years ago to the advent of agriculture some 10,000–12,000 years ago. So, for the better part of human existence, grains did not comprise any notable portion of the human diet. In essence, what has become the bulk of our modern diet was missing from the diet of our prehistoric ancestors.

5. Grains aren't good for your joints.

Due to their inflammatory nature, grains – even whole grains – are linked to joint pain and arthritis.
Grains' amino acid composition mirrors that of the soft tissue in your joints. Because both synovial tissue and grains are chemically similar, your body has difficulty differentiating between the two. So, when your immune cells get all hot and bothered by inflammation caused by grain and begin to attack it as a foreign invader, they also begin to attack the soft tissue in your joint – leading to pain, autoimmune diseases like rheumatoid arthritis and, of course, more inflammation.

6. Poorly prepared grains prevent mineral absorption.

When improperly prepared, as they most often are, grains can inhibit vitamin and mineral absorption. Grains contain substances like phytic acid which binds up minerals and prevents proper absorption. Essentially, though your diet might be rich in iron, calcium and other vital nutrients if you eat improperly prepared grain, you're not fully absorbing nutrients from the foods you eat.

7. Grains are bad for your teeth.

Due to those high levels of phytates in grain, grain

is linked to dental decay. With high levels of mineral-blocking phytic acid coupled with low mineral absorption rates and plenty of starches for bacteria to feed on, grain contributes to dental decay.

8. Grains aren't good for your skin either.

Grains have a very high carbohydrate content and while the carbohydrates in grain are complex, they are still broken down into sugars nonetheless. These sugars instruct your body to produce more insulin and insulin-like growth factor (IFG-1). Elevated insulin levels lead to a cascading hormonal response and these hormones activate the sebum-producing glands in your skin – encouraging them to produce more oil. IFG-1 is also linked with increased production of keratinocytes which also contribute to acne.

9. Eating grain makes you crave grain.

Foods rich in carbohydrates give you quick energy, but that energy wears off just as quickly as it came. Since grains break down into sugar, they create a rise in insulin levels. When those levels fall, you crave more.

In this section, I would like to share some cases that you can follow through with me to see how I treated each patient.

Ellen

Ellen came to my office complaining of fatigue, lack of energy and weight gain. Her doctor had her on thyroid medication, cholesterol medication and Vitamin D.

I reviewed her most recent lab results and ordered a comprehensive blood panel which includes the tests I outlined in Chapter 4. Surprisingly, the most glaring finding was that Ellen's blood sugar was 118. I say surprisingly because Ellen suspected her problem was with her thyroid and that is why she was on thyroid medication. We also ordered food sensitivity testing to allow us to formulate a diet for Ellen.

We began by placing Ellen on a diet that consisted of mainly fruits, meats and vegetable. She started supplementing Omega 3 fatty acids and Glysen from Apex. We also added some probiotics and gut repair protocols. Within a month, Ellen's energy levels started to improve dramatically. With this new found energy, she started to use her body more. She lost 15 lbs. in 2 months. After one year, Ellen has lost a total of 40 lbs. and her energy is excellent. Her doctor has taken her off cholesterol medication and reduced her thyroid medication. The key in this case was recognizing that the solution was correcting the blood sugar problem.

Amoura

Amoura's two major complaints were extreme fatigue and weight gain. She had been on every diet imaginable and all without success. Her energy levels dragged all day long. Her medication was Synthroid and cholesterol medication. Her initial blood tests revealed that Amoura was positive for Hashimoto's (her TPO antibodies were out of range). In addition, her total T3 levels were also low at 65. (Functional normal is 110-180). We ran food sensitivity tests that showed she had sensitivities to gluten, coffee, dairy and soy. We began with one month gut repair (GI Revive) and Vitamin D, glutathione and Omega 3 fatty acids. After 2 weeks, we added a dose of 100 billion probiotic. She also followed the autoimmune diet. After the first month we added some B vitamins to support the liver and to improve conversion of T4 to T3 in that area. We also suggested Amoura consult with her primary care physician in regards to the low T3 level. Her doctor switched her medication to Cytomel. After 12 weeks, Amoura lost over 15 lbs. and she is full of energy.

Kathy

Kathy's main complaints were low energy, hair loss, weight gain, body aches and joint pain, anxiety and depression. She had a history of goiter and elevated antibodies testing positive for Hashimoto's. Kathy had been working with an alternative doctor that was helping her with her hormones and was also on a diet that was mostly fruits and vegetables. She was 62 years old and for the most part took very good care of herself in regard to diet and nutrition. She was frustrated that her efforts were not helping her at all. We ran complete bloodwork, adrenal tests and ELISA ACT food tests. Even though Kathy's diet was very clean, she tested positive for chicken, clam, milk, okra, olive, plum and sorghum.

Thyroid testing showed a TSH of 4.71 (functional normal is 1.8-3.0), a T4 of 6 (6-12), a Total T3 of 79 (100-180), T3 uptake 30 (28-38) and reverse T3 of 16 (7-24). Protein was 6.7 (6.9-7.4), Globulin was 2.2 (2.4-2.8) indicating hypochlorhydria (low stomach acid).

In this case, thyroid function was not ideal and the cause was the autoimmune attack on the thyroid. We went a step further to measure ideal thyroid function and applied the Total T3 and reverse T3 ratio. Total T3 divided by reverse T3 should be 10 or greater. Kathy's result was 79/16 = 4.9.

Vitamin D levels were 79 which is perfect for someone with autoimmune disease.

Kathy's history also indicated an issue with her adrenal glands as she stated she was diagnosed with a congenital disease affecting the adrenals. We performed an adrenal stress test. Results showed normal cortisol production and DHEA - which was surprising.

With Kathy, we started by balancing her immune system with Apex products and addressed leaky gut along with probiotics. We also added B vitamins to help with converting T4 to T3. We modified her diet so as to eliminate the food sensitivities we found. Lastly, we used Xeneplex to help detox the liver. After the final step, Kathy finally began to notice that she was feeling better than she had in years. We also assisted the thyroid with Thyroven from PRL.

Eight months later, her new thyroid panel showed Total T3 at 112, reverse T3 at 9.8, T4 at 7. The Total T3/reverse T3 ratio was now 11.2

Most importantly, Kathy was feeling much better. Her energy levels were back to normal, body aches have disappeared, hair loss stopped and weight became manageable. Kathy was taking Naturethroid as prescribed by her doctor.

Janet G.

Janet came to see me because she wanted someone that could help her with Hashimoto's. She complained of fatigue and weight gain. She had previously consulted with an alternative practitioner and was on numerous supplements to help the adrenal glands and Iodine to help the thyroid. She became alarmed when she noticed that her thyroid gland had been enlarging and stopped taking her supplements.

We ran food sensitivity testing that showed reactions to grapes, lemon, salmon, avocado, tapioca, and bay leaf. Stool testing showed an overgrowth of yeast. Adrenal gland testing showed Cortisol levels and rhythm to be normal. However, her DHEA level was depleted at 1.0 (normal is 2.0-10.0). Her thyroid panel was within normal limits and we tested her TPO and thyroglobulin antibodies and confirmed they were high, indicating Hashimoto's.

With Janet, we modified her diet and eliminated sensitivities. We put her on DHEA and supplements to help balance her immune system. As we progressed, we also used some natural products for yeast from Apex. Once we had her digestive tract clean, we performed a Vitamin C flush and detox.

After 6 months, her energy levels are normal and she had lost 12 lbs. She feels fantastic and believes she has her health under control.

As far as the thyroid gland enlarging, Janet had a biopsy performed and it showed that malignant cells were found. She had surgery to remove only the cancerous parts. Today, her thyroid works perfectly as her blood tests show. Janet is not on any thyroid medication.

Mellisa A.

Mellisa was in college and constantly complained of weight gain and low energy. She was born with a congenitally small thyroid and had been on Synthroid since birth. She and her doctor struggled to get her TSH normal.

Blood tests showed that Melissa was iron deficient as her iron levels were low and her ferritin was 6 (norm 10-122).

Adrenal testing showed depleted Cortisol in the morning at 7 (normal 13-24). Mellisa did not have Hashimoto's.

We changed Mellissa's eating habits as she ate infrequently and usually skipped breakfast. Her diet was a Paleo diet free of gluten. This was not an easy task as Mellisa lived on campus and was limited to her food choices. Nevertheless, we managed to help with basically eliminating as much as we could. We should also mention that Mellisa was on birth control pills, which meant that we needed to support the liver pathways to help clear hormone.

We supplemented an HCl product from Apex along with Vitamin C to help with iron absorption. We also added a vegetarian based iron supplement to help increase depleted levels. In addition, we aggressively supplemented with adrenal supplement to increase morning Cortisol levels.

After four months, Mellisa had lost 20 pounds and her energy levels improved. Her TSH level was finally normal and her ferritin (iron) level began to climb. She ended up writing a paper on the Paleo diet.

The patients that have the greatest success are those that have the motivation and discipline to follow through. Our body changes approximately every seven days. And thus, you are creating new function roughly every seven days. To naturally get your body working more efficiently, it could very well take 6-18 months or longer. However, many patients can start to feel better within just a few weeks or months! I usually work with patients for a period of 36 months and most of them are feeling 70-100% better.

If you're looking for someone to help guide you personally or have any questions, feel free to contact me:

Dr Tom Sladic

thenaturalthyroiddoctor.com

69352442R00068

Made in the USA
Lexington, KY
29 October 2017